Mary Ellen's
Help Yourself
Diet Plan

Mary Ellen's Help Yourself *Diet Plan*

"The one that worked for me"

by Mary Ellen Pinkham

Foreword by Joel S. Holger, M.D.

St. Martin's / Marek
New York

This book is dedicated to
Sherman F. Pinkham, Jr., the man I live with,
and Jonathon Lazear, the man I work with.

Grateful acknowledgment is made for permission to abridge the listing on page 165 from pages 154–155 in *Food Values of Portions Commonly Used*, Thirteenth Edition by Jean A. T. Pennington and Helen Nichols Church. Copyright © 1980 by Helen Nichols Church, B.S., and Jean A. T. Pennington, Ph.D., R.D. Reprinted by permission of Harper & Row, Publishers, Inc.

Design by M. Paul

Library of Congress Cataloging in Publication Data

Pinkham, Mary Ellen.
    Mary Ellen's help yourself diet plan.

    "A St. Martin's Press/Marek book."

    Includes index.
    1. Reducing diets. I. Title.
RM222.2.P56   1983   613.2′5   82-21572
ISBN 0-312-51863-3

10 9 8 7 6 5 4 3

CONTENTS

Acknowledgments   viii

Foreword by Joel S. Holger, M.D.   ix

Introduction   xi

Part One
Help Wanted: My Story

Chapter 1
The Gang of One   2

Chapter 2
A Fat Madness   8

Chapter 3
The Hippy Housewife   13

Chapter 4
Success Went to My Waistline   19

Chapter 5
Facing the Fat Facts   25

Chapter 6
What's Up, Doc?   31

Chapter 7
The Moving Experience   38

Chapter 8
When the Compliments Stop   45

Chapter 9
Fat No More   51

Part Two
Help Yourself: The Program

Chapter 10
If You Really Want to Help Yourself,
Read This Part   56

Chapter 11
Now That You're Ready to Choose
Your Own Menus . . .   90

Chapter 12
The Walkout—Easier Than a Workout   107

Chapter 13
Mary Ellen's Forty-four Best Diet Tips   121

Part Three
Second Helpings

Chapter 14
Nibbles   139

Chapter 15
Q&A   144

Chapter 16
Fact/Fiction   148

Chapter 17
Did You Know That? . . .   152

Chapter 18
The Most Dangerous Things to Put in Your Mouth   158

Chapter 19
Formerly Fattening Recipes   177

Chapter 20
Alternatives and Substitutes: Or, How to
Eat an Egg Without Eating an Egg   190

Chapter 21
Seasonal Guide to Dieter's Dilemmas   194

Chapter 22
Other Ways to Fry a Fish   197

Chapter 23
A Pat on Your (Thin) Back   200

Chapter 24
A Note About Calorie Counters   202

    Diet Diary   206
    A Final Thought   207
    Index   208

ACKNOWLEDGMENTS

I'd like to acknowledge the help of lots and lots of people, but I've been told I've only got room here for a few. I'd like to single out for thanks:

Dale Burg, my collaborator and sounding board, whose help and support saw me through this project. She's the best!

Dr. Joel Holger, my internist, a wonderful find: a man who knows his ABC's—and a few other important letters—in the nutrition field. I want to thank him for his guidance and patience.

Judith C. Goldberg, nutritionist extraordinaire, whose doctoral work was in the area of obesity. Judy helped me out in every phase of this project. She's some smart cookie!

C. B. Abbott, whose research was great. When several nutritionists saw the material Connie dug up, they were amazed. The CIA would be lucky to have a researcher like her.

Walter C. Hewett, an ex-chronic dieter, now a weight counselor. Walter finally came to grips with everything that chronic dieting entails and wound up a good (and thin) advisor and example.

Samuel Kaplan, my lawyer. He's my friend, too. Everyone on earth should have that combo, but not everyone is as lucky as I am. He supported me all the way.

Tom Oberg, George Cleveland, Kathy Rice, and Wendy Lazear, members of the Mary Ellen Enterprises staff. Behind the scenes, they helped in many ways and were always there for me.

Andrew Pinkham, my son. When he told his mom she reminded him of the fat little mouse in *Cinderella*, he sure started something. . . .

FOREWORD

I've already offered my congratulations to Mary Ellen Pinkham—the new Mary Ellen Pinkham, nearly eighty pounds leaner and more fit than when I first met her. Now I congratulate you for starting this book. I am sure you'll find it a treat to read, and I think it contains more than a few surprises. This book can change your life, if you let it.

When Mary Ellen came to us, she was complaining of the flu: She was tired, worn out, and feverish. But even before she'd become ill, she hadn't felt well. She was significantly overweight and tired of constant dieting without much result.

She told me that she'd been on one diet or another for as long as she could remember—all failures. She didn't realize, until I told her, that was the key to her problem. She was a victim of dieting. Fad dieting had changed her metabolism so that she could never hope to lose weight and keep it off.

My practice is not oriented toward the treatment of obesity, but as an internist I estimate that nearly half my patients are concerned about being too overweight. Rarely does a day go by without a patient asking my advice about diets or dieting. And, often, the stories I hear are similar to Mary Ellen's. The patient has lost weight on diet after diet, then regained it all and often a few extra pounds.

It seemed to me that there were certain basic, scientific principles that most dieters were failing to take into account. It further seemed possible to devise a program that incorporated these principles.

When I got to know Mary Ellen a little better and we discussed the extent of her problem, she was very excited by the information I shared with her. She said she felt that was the first time she really got the truth about diets and dieting.

What I explained to her was not difficult to understand, but it was up to her to put the ideas into effect once we'd worked out a plan, for we agreed she would be the subject to prove the findings of current research. Together, we found ways to help Mary Ellen change her metabolism and get rid of inappropriate eating habits. As soon as she began to get results, Mary Ellen made the commitment to follow through and the ultimate promise to herself that she would adhere to this new way of living on a life-long basis.

What follows is the story of Mary Ellen's experience and the plan that worked for her. You'll enjoy it, because everyone likes to read a successful story. What you should especially enjoy is the knowledge that her success can be duplicated by others. The plan, in theory, cannot fail; but it does demand work. I hope you try it. And I hope you find it's not only the one that worked for Mary Ellen but also the one that works for you.

Joel S. Holger, M.D.
Minneapolis, Minnesota
September 30, 1982

INTRODUCTION

I'm in the business of solving problems, and I'm pretty good at what I do. Reading my mail makes me proud. "Dear Mary Ellen, You helped me solve a problem nobody else could."

But looking in my mirror brought me down. I was a problem solver with a very big problem—a problem I'd been fighting for years. My weight.

For years I struggled with it. For a while I decided to live with it.

Then, in January 1982, something finally snapped. It was the band on my maternity half-slip, the one I reserved to wear when I was feeling fat. Feeling fat? I *was* fat. Who was I trying to kid? I was telling the salesladies I needed the larger sizes because I'd recently had a baby. The fact was that "baby" was already reading the newspapers. I hadn't been pregnant in seven years. Now I had had it.

I was ready to start my last diet—the one that worked. It had to be different from all the ones I'd tried before. I found it, and it worked for me. I'd like to share my diet plan, and my story, with you. I think you'll probably find some of it is your story, too. Maybe we can share the same happy ending.

Part One

Help Wanted: My Story

Chapter 1

The Gang of One

Among the souvenirs of my childhood, along with a diary into which I had taped my first underarm hair and a letter with Elvis Presley's rubber-stamped signature declining my dinner invitation, is a certificate from the Minnesota Girl Scouts Association. It testifies that in 1957 I sold more Girl Scout cookies than any other girl in the green-uniformed ranks.

Everyone wanted to know how I did it. Here's the true story: I was my own best customer. You know the old line, "What are little girls made of?" In the winter of 1957, my body composition was probably about half chocolate mint Girl Scout cookies.

Things were never the same after that. Oh, the input varied. You know how the Chinese have the Year of the Dog, the Year of the Dragon, and so forth? I had my years, too. After the Year of the Chocolate Mint Cookies, I had the Year of Burger and Fries, the Year of the Big Mac, and the Year of the Tuna Melt. The melody would change, but the theme remained the same.

For most of my life, I had a weight problem. Now I don't. I assume if you're reading this book, it's because you have a weight problem, too. Actually, what you have is a fat problem—but I'll explain that later. The point is that you don't feel comfortable with the way you are.

Now, I had a *major* fat problem. Anything over fifty pounds, you have to admit, is a major fat problem. But friends with far less than that to lose tell me that their weight—or their fat—is just as big a problem for them as mine was for me. Carrying around even a few extra pounds, they say, makes them unhappy: Their clothes don't feel right and they're very uncomfortable.

Feeling fat affects every stage of your life. Where you work. Where you vacation. Whom you end up marrying. How you raise your kids.

My profession has been influenced by my fat. Believe it or not, I have a fairly nice singing voice. And I really believe that if weight hadn't been an obstacle in my life, today I might be a singer. But I always felt: Mary Ellen, you've got to lose the weight before you audition. (Of course, this never stopped Pavarotti, but then they don't write roles like Salome for men.)

You may have had the same attitude yourself: I'm not going to apply for the job of my choice until I'm down to my goal weight. I won't find the man of my dreams until I'm at my goal weight; in fact, I won't even feel comfortable about any guy who's attracted to me now, because after all, what kind of man would like a heavy woman? Now, whether or not this kind of thinking is good for you is a matter of debate, but the point is that in this society, it's very hard to feel good about yourself unless you're lean and fit.

You miss out on an awful lot. After my first book was published and turned out to be a success, the natural thing would have been to treat myself and my family to a little vacation, right? Wrong. Vacations to most people, and to me, mean beaches, and beaches mean bathing suits. Dressed, I was a successful author. In a bathing suit, I was, well, let's put it this way: No beach coverup manufactured would do the job I wanted.

Actually, I didn't start out in life with a major weight problem. I was a curly-headed baby. People in my family said I looked like a Korean War orphan, but obviously they didn't know what they were talking about because at eight pounds I was a little hefty to fit that description. Granted, that's not what you might call a mammoth child, especially since I was a month overdue, but it's definitely on the large end of the baby scale. I must have enjoyed food right from the beginning because I actually remember first tasting solid foods. It was an experience I can't really explain—remember, it happened before I knew words—but I do remember that it was heavenly.

When you're the first child, with a loving, caring mother, you're fed very well. I certainly was. By the time I was in sixth grade, she was already concerned that I might become overweight. I don't believe in kids going on diets. I admire parents who don't nag their kids about weight. The problem will go away if their diets are nutritious and they get exercise. Of course, people are much more conscious of weight than when I was a child. In those days, people thought the Campbell kids were cute because they had such round cheeks. Now everyone wants to have a Dannon body.

3

When I began my diet, I set a goal weight of 135 pounds. That's about fifteen pounds less than Venus de Milo would have weighed, with arms, if she'd been made of flesh instead of stone, according to an article I once read. It's what I weighed at sixteen. I wasn't a beanpole, but I was at a good weight, and I was in shape.

It's generally accepted that your teenage weight, if you weren't a chubbette, is the right weight for you as an adult. That should be your goal weight on this diet. If you can't remember what you weighed, try and check out old medical records. Of course, if you're like most of us who've been dieting for most of our lives, you probably do remember.

My friend Gail, an addicted dieter like me, says that while other people remember where they were on certain important dates, she remembers what she weighed. She knows that when Neil Armstrong landed on the moon she was down to 125.

I'm not the only one who has gained weight since my teenage years. The whole country has gotten fatter. I was just doing the American thing. Yes. You may be surprised to hear this, but over the past fifteen years, Americans as a whole have gained weight while eating less.

I'm certainly eating less than I used to. I'm from a Swedish background, and the Swedes eat a pretty hearty diet. My grandfather was a butcher. My mother wrote a little poem that I used to recite.

> My grandfather is a butcher,
> My mother cuts the meat,
> And I am a little rump roast,
> Running down the street.

Ultimately, my grandmother did more of the meat cutting than my mother, since my mother was out working. My grandmother is your typical wonderful, soft, chubby, loving grandmother, and she loved to cook for me and my sister and brother. My favorite of the lunches she prepared was peanut butter and tapioca pudding. After I ate the peanut butter sandwich, I'd have a couple of bowls of pudding. I'd already had my oatmeal and bacon in the morning, of course, and I would be ready for meat and potato and vegetable for dinner.

My grandmother also baked. She made cake doughnuts and raised doughnuts, and after they were fried she sprinkled sugar on them. She wouldn't just give us one or two, she'd give us ten. (I'd hide mine so nobody could get them.) But this was a special event. We didn't get dessert and cakes and cookies the way you can today. Cake wasn't a daily item on the menu, it was a weekly treat. If you wanted a cake, you didn't get it in the stores; you made a scratch cake. I think if we still had to prepare all our food from scratch, we'd have less of a national weight problem. By the time you get out the pan, beater, flour, and sugar and then discover you're out of vanilla—the urge has probably passed. But you could have eaten a box of cookies in the same amount of time.

Also, have you noticed the national gain in weight is coinciding with the decline in the size of the family? Don't laugh, folks: I think they're related. In the old days, when you divided your cake with the family, you only got one slice. Today, with smaller households, there are three people sharing cakes that used to be divided by six. They're eating twice as much. Also, of course, we didn't have fast foods back then.

What we did have, I was eating. And a lot of it. Still, I wasn't fat, just what they call sturdy. Whatever I ate, I burned up. I never stopped moving. First of all, I didn't even remember seeing a school bus when I was a kid. We walked to school, at least three miles a day. After school, we were constantly in the streets playing kick-the-can and baseball. And we had chores. On Saturdays, first we cut the lawns with hand mowers, and then we worked off more energy jumping up and down whenever we stepped in the dog-doo, which happened at least once every Saturday. In the fall, we raked leaves into piles, and then we had to jump in the piles, and then we had to rake the leaves all over again. In the winter, which lasts quite a while in Minnesota, we shoveled snow. And after that we had to make a snowman.

We had housekeeping chores, too. When I was growing up, it was my responsibility to iron my own clothes. And that's when I believe my hinting career started. In those days, everything was cotton, and you know how wrinkled cotton gets after it's been laundered. What we did was sprinkle the clothes with water, roll them up, put them in plastic bags, and store them in the refrigerator for a couple of hours. This made the ironing chore much easier.

Well, I had lots of other things I would rather do than iron, so sometimes I'd let the ironing go for a couple of days. By the time I got around to my clothes, I'd take them out of the refrigerator and find that they had mildew all over them.

Eventually, the light bulb went off in my head: I'd freeze the clothes. That way I could iron one piece at a time. Of course, we didn't have big freezers in those days, just those little compartments, so there would be several items of my wardrobe stuffed into the spaces where the ice cubes should have been. I was always getting yelled at. "Mary Ellen, get down here and get your peasant blouse out of the freezer."

Even when we watched TV we had to move at least a little. As some of you may remember, in those days you actually had to get up and go over to the set to change the channel. In fact, we didn't watch much TV, and my mother always got rid of the television set in the summer. For some reason, it always managed to go on the blink the week school let out. But we had plenty to do without it. Minnesota is the land of 10,000 lakes, and just four blocks from my home were four of them. They were like private playgrounds for us kids.

For my first twelve years I was a tomboy, involved in everything from climbing trees to stealing apples. Then I discovered boys.

When I became a young teenager, inactivity was voguish. If you were lucky enough to hang around with a group in which somebody had a car, you were really popular. You didn't walk anyplace, and you wouldn't be caught dead on a bike. Only the simps rode their bikes to school.

Looking good ruled out any physical activity—those cotton clothes really wrinkled. We didn't have miracle fibers. Today, you can slip into a pair of polyester pants in the morning, go stunt riding all day, and the pants won't show a crease. Back then, the minute you bent over, you were a mess.

And the hairstyles! Hair was tortured into place. You sat under the dryer for hours or you slept in rollers. It's amazing we don't all have permanent furrows in our scalp. I wore medium-sized rollers, which meant my head never got nearer than two inches from the pillow. My best friend set her hair around orange juice cans and slept sitting up. In the morning, you'd take out the rollers and shoot a lot of spray net over the whole thing. The desired effect was that your hair looked bulletproof. Someone told me my hair looked like fake Dynel and I took that as a compliment because that meant it must have looked really neat. Anyone who wanted to look good knew you had to move around slowly, so you wouldn't ruin your clothes or disturb your hair.

Until this time, I'd done all right in gym. I was a great

basketball player, and I was good at running and jumping. I'd always felt a little inadequate because I couldn't climb the ropes, but at this point I really started to hate gym class. It was partly because of the group showers. They never upset me so much that I'd hide in my locker, but I was modest, and besides, I was worried about my hair. Here I was at the time of my life when looks are the most important thing in the world, and someone expected me to go to gym class in the second period to do a hundred situps and then get my hair wet on top of it.

It became a big game to get out of going to gym. I was at my most ingenious each spring, when we'd have to do these crazy marathon runs. Mind you, we did not run all winter long, but for some reason the gym teacher thought it would be fun to send us to run four miles the minute she saw a crocus. Of course, today they know this kind of thing could kill a person. But there we were.

I had a few friends who'd graduated, and I called on them for help. I'd start off from the school and go maybe a quarter of a mile. Then my friends would pick me up in someone's beat-up old convertible with the top down—it was spring, after all—and we'd go to Porky's, the local drive-in. We'd all have a Coke and then they'd drop me off a block from school and I'd come in with a fairly reasonable run. I never tried to set any kind of record, because I knew the teacher would figure that one out.

Even though I didn't move around as much when I became a teenager, I still had my former appetite. Gradually I started gaining weight. And I didn't know why. I really, truly, didn't know why. I started cutting back like a typical teenager—going to the diner for a burger, fries, and a Coke once a day, and then picking all the rest of the day. I never had a major weight problem—but I never got any thinner, either.

So the vicious cycle began.

Chapter 2

A Fat Madness

I turned on the television one day and two doctors were talking about when diets began. This was an intriguing idea to me, that somebody could pin a date on the whole thing. The experts couldn't narrow it down to a year, but they agreed that fad diets really caught on big in the early 1950s.

I do know that in 1959 a group of friends and I went on the Minneapolis diet. The Minneapolis diet, which we made up, was as follows:

Monday
Coca-Cola (all you want)
Pistachio nuts (all you want)

The program was the same for Tuesday, Wednesday, Thursday, Friday, Saturday, and Sunday. We arrived at pistachio nuts because we decided we were going to eat only one food, so it should be something we liked, and we all liked pistachio nuts.

The Minneapolis diet had two features I always looked for in diets afterward: "Fast weight loss" and "Eat all you want." Those were the attractions of the first official diet I went on, something that later became known as Dr. Atkins' diet. (When it first appeared, Dr. Atkins was probably just finishing up his residency.) The diet was explained in a book called *Calories Don't Count*, and at the time I believed that. After all, who'd ever seen a calorie?

The *Calories Don't Count* diet was a low carbohydrate diet. From health class I knew all foods were made of protein, fat, or carbohydrate, and I bought a book that gave the carbohydrate count of common foods so I could avoid those that were high in carbohydrates. Still, I had to have my Coca-Cola, even though that used up half my carbohydrate allowance for the day. I starved, and I lost weight. Temporarily.

I went back on that diet when it came out under Dr. Atkins' name. I followed Dr. Stillman's diet, too. Remember that one? You ate a lot of protein and drank a lot of water. An enormous amount of water. With the obvious results. It was definitely not a diet you'd recommend to someone who, for example, collected tolls on the New Jersey Turnpike.

I liked it because you could eat all the meat you wanted to, any kind. My version of the Stillman diet was four pork chops and a gallon of water for dinner. I lost a lot of weight in a single weekend and put it back on the following weekend.

In basic health class, you learn that the body is supposed to be in a state of balance. Everything that goes in and out is supposed to maintain that balance. On the "miracle" diets, you send the system into a tailspin.

There are many variations of those high protein or high fat, low carbohydrate diets. The secret weapon is ketosis. The theory is that protein molecules are so large and complex that they require more energy to digest, and you can burn extra calories every day just by eating extra protein. Supposedly, you also eventually excrete a byproduct of fat metabolism (called ketone bodies) that contains undigested calories. The latest news is that the maximum calories you can excrete in this fashion is only a hundred! Besides, the side effects of these diets are nausea, weakness, lightheadedness, and fatigue. You also break down your muscles and weaken your bones, and on top of everything else, you get bad breath. I was led to believe that the worse your breath smelled, the more weight you were losing. As if I didn't have enough problems.

I found the vinegar and honey diet floating around somewhere in the sixties. Honey and vinegar was mixed with warm water and a glassful was drunk before each meal. If you've read my other books you know I'm the expert on vinegar. On this diet, the only thing you were guaranteed to lose were your teeth. I didn't stay on it long.

Diets named after foods became very popular about then. I went on all of them. I couldn't wait for the latest women's magazine to come out and tell me about the newest diet. I went on the cottage cheese diet, the apple diet, and the grape diet. I even made up one of my own. It was called the sauerkraut diet. I figured that anything tasting that terrible would surely burn off fat. (In those days, I was always hoping to "burn off" fat. Nobody told me that was a laugh.)

Guess what I found out? There is not a canned food on the market that has more salt in it than sauerkraut. If you know anything about salt, you can imagine that not much weight loss occurred on this diet. I just really hate sauerkraut now.

My girlfriend Melissa had a little more success with her own Arch and Box diet. It was a fast food program. For one week she took all her meals at McDonald's and Jack in the Box. She'd get up in the morning and drive over to get some Eggs McMuffin and then around lunchtime she'd buy the Box special—burger and fries. Of course, by the end of the week, she'd gotten pretty tired of burgers and fries, so she'd indirectly cut her caloric intake. She lost five pounds, which she kept off for about five days.

Meanwhile, I was on the grapefruit diet, which meant I drank a lot of grapefruit juice before each meal. (Why? It burned off the fat, of course.) And then you ate one egg, with one slice of bacon. If you had two eggs, you had two slices of bacon. If you had three eggs, you had three slices of bacon. I liked the bacon, but the rules were very clear: If you ate four slices of bacon, you ate four eggs.

Later on, I put two and two together and realized this diet was probably a plot of the American Poultry Association! At the time, I was happy with it, since I lost weight.

By the time I'd gained it back, I'd heard about the Mayo Clinic diet. The Mayo Clinic refused to take the rap for this diet, probably because the diet also originated with the American Poultry Association. On this diet, you ate two eggs with every meal. Egg yolks, in addition to having 60 calories each, are loaded with cholesterol. (And they don't burn fat.) At the time, I was ignorant of this fact. I thought the diet was great and went on it frequently.

Until, that is, I discovered the Alpine Ski diet. This was similar to the Mayo Clinic diet, but instead of two eggs, you had one. Actually, you had two in the morning and then only one at lunch and one at dinner. Why it was called the Alpine Ski diet I never did figure out. Maybe it was started by the Swiss Poultry Association.

What all these diets had in common was that you were always deprived of something. By "something," I don't mean obvious no-nos like cake and cookies, but foods that are part of most people's daily routine. On some, you aren't even allowed to eat fruit. I'm not especially fond of fruit, but tell me I can't eat it and I'm ready to kill for strawberries and apples. That's why I never lasted longer than two weeks on any diet.

Naturally, I was attracted to diets that made me think I would not be deprived. Authors had people like me in mind when they started bringing out diet books that made the whole process seem like fun: *The Drinking Man's Diet. Eat, Drink, and Get Thin. Stuff Your Way to Svelteness. Pig Out and Pare Down.* Who do you think was first in line at the bookstore?

I went on every diet ever set in print and several that were passed along in the oral (how appropriate) tradition. For example, the bowl diet invented by my friend Marcia. On the bowl diet, you select your size bowl, and then fill it three times a day with anything you like. But you can only fill it once per meal. The theory is that you might eat ice cream, but you wouldn't put a steak and ice cream in the bowl together. Oh, yeah?

Sandy told me about her three-food diet: Select any three foods that have nutritional value and eat them for a week. For one of my foods, I selected "deli." I took in so much grease that if I walked barefoot, I tended to skid. Plus I gained weight. Bambi told me *her* magic formula: She made it a rule to eat *only* the specific food she wanted at a particular moment, the more exotic the better. In other words, if she had a yen for veal parmigiana, she had to find a restaurant where it was served. The idea was that the longer it took you to find the food you were in search of, the longer the time period when you weren't eating at all. This was a great idea in the days when exotic foods were harder to get, when the only people who ever heard of, say, Mexican food, were Mexicans. Today, you can get an enchilada in the middle of nowhere.

I was going up and down on these diets for years. If I wasn't gaining weight, I was on a diet. When I dieted, I would read cookbooks. My friends would call and I'd say, "Can I get back to you? I'm in the middle of a good part." Eventually I went on a new diet every night, not even waiting for Mondays.

You're going to ask why I didn't go to a doctor. Well, most of them had been unsympathetic to my problem. One told me not to bother to come back until I'd lost twenty pounds. Another greeted me by saying, "Hmmm. This looks like a beef trust." Not only did I not like dieting, I didn't want to face a scale.

Then I heard of a doctor who didn't weigh you: He just measured you. He had a thick German accent and I think he was en route to Argentina when he ran out of money in Minneapolis. He gave daily injections of something extracted, from what I could gather, from the urine of pregnant cows. That alone should have made his patients lose their appetites, but in case they didn't, they were also under strict orders not to eat more than two small portions of meat and vegetables twice a day. No one ate very much under his

11

care, but they all thought the "magic" injections did the trick.

If I didn't want to see him, I could have gone to Harriet's diet doctor. She'd been with him for fifteen years. He's in Manhattan, and so is she, but he thought she lived in Philadelphia. That's because he charges $250 a year to see local patients, but only $15 a month to people from out of town. She'd call up and say, "Hi, doc, it's me, Harriet, calling long distance." She wanted to have a record of the Liberty Bell ringing to play in the background until I told her that *it* was cracked, too.

I rejected both those solutions and went to see Alice's diet doctor instead. Well, I didn't actually see him: You had to lose twenty pounds before you could see him. Meanwhile, you were seen by one of his associates, who sat in small cubicles under laminated plaques of their medical degrees and dispensed large quantities of pills in various colors. In a laughable attempt to appear legitimate, the cubicle doctors took your blood pressure when you came in.

The pills were vitamins and speed. They worked for a while, but soon I became immune to them. Eventually, they just made me eat faster. I also vacuumed a lot and called people I hadn't seen in years. When I came down off the pills, I found myself booked for numerous lunch dates with people I barely remembered. I also made lists— such as whom I'd invite to a party in five years and the clothes I planned to buy in 1995.

Several years ago, my friend Sandy in Los Angeles invited me to see her doctor. He had his nurse touch the patient, and he touched the nurse, and this way he got emanations that would tell him what foods Sandy was allergic to. If she stopped eating them, he said, she would lose weight. He also told her she would lose weight if she wore green. "That's crazy," she told him. "Try it," he said.

Before I had a chance to decide whether to fly out and see that one, Sandy found one she swore was even better—a chiropractor-nutritionist, a dual specialty that seems to be popular in Los Angeles. The doctors out there get crazier the nearer their offices are to the beach, and this one was in Pacific Palisades. He specialized in food allergies, too, and his method involved applying foods to your body to see which ones you are allergic to. The way I pictured it, he'd put fudge on your forearm and asparagus on your abdomen, and from that he'd figure out your story.

He never got to do anything with my abdomen, though. My gynecologist got there first. He told me I was pregnant.

Chapter 3

The Hippy Housewife

I was twenty-nine when I became pregnant. I'd been married for six years. I thought of myself as a sweet little June bride, but actually I got married in March. Fortunately, the snow didn't interfere with the ceremony, since I had planned on a small wedding. For some reason, I was self-conscious. Though I would eventually do television shows without any anxiety, I felt uncomfortable about having an audience watch me get married. After the ceremony, the wedding party went out to celebrate in a restaurant (where else?).

I weighed about 130 on our wedding day. I'd gotten my weight down to even a little lower than that, but the popping of the question seemed destined to be followed by the popping of my seams.

I thought of my high school friend Gail, who each year went off her diet the minute someone asked her to the prom. Once you hook the guy, she explained, it was okay to start eating again.

At 130, people tell me, I was looking good. I wasn't happy at that weight, though. Until I finished the Help Yourself diet, I can't remember a time when I was happy with my body. I think that's a problem many fat people have. They fall off the diet wagon because they're not satisfied, even when they've reached their goal weight. They don't believe that they're thin enough. I read about a study in which people drew pictures of themselves at the beginning of a diet and then at the end. At the beginning, they always draw themselves looking thinner than they are, and at the end, they always draw themselves larger. It takes a while to develop the proper self-image. Anyway, there I was, unhappy at 130. I vowed that the number on the scale would change. It did—to 160. I shot up thirty pounds within six months, and there I stayed.

Actually, people tell me I didn't look bad at that weight, either. But no one went so far as to say I looked great. I'm not sure how the weight gain happened. Of course, I was eating a lot of steak. For those who have never tasted it, I just have to tell you a little about pan-fried steak. You take a steak and cut the fat off. Then you pound the steak with a hammer to flatten it. Then you heat a fry pan until it's red hot, throw the fat in till it melts a little, and throw in the steak. (I hope that didn't trigger anybody who's reading this to go right in the kitchen, but I think the recipe's too good not to share. Pass it along to your thin friends.) Anyway, I can probably attribute some of my early marriage weight gain to pan-fried steak.

The weight didn't bother Sherm. He always told me he thought I was attractive. And I want it understood that I'm not putting any guilt trip on him, but often the people you love help contribute to your problem. For example, I might have been eating pretty sensibly for the week, then all of a sudden I'd get an urge for ice cream, which is not unreasonable. Even thin people get urges for certain foods. But I was overweight, and you can't really binge when you're overweight and you aren't moving around.

Anyway, Sherm would go up to the store and bring home the ice cream, and he'd have a little dish. I'd have a bowlful. Or two. After eating, I always said, "Don't ever do that again," and once he realized what I was talking about, he'd say he wouldn't. Then I would say, "Now, look, you have to promise me. If I tell you to go over to the White Castle and pick up some burgers, tell me no."

But I could always talk him into it. Sherm is a normal person. He didn't see anything wrong with eating ice cream or burgers. He thinks like a normal person, in singles, not multiples: one burger, not a sackful, one dish of ice cream, not a bowl.

I remember seeing a Jules Feiffer cartoon that was a strip of panels. Each picture had the same woman in it, and she had the same long face in each. In the first panel, she's saying, "I keep thinking my life would be better if I were married," and then in the next one, she's saying, "I would have a better job if I were married," and "I would live in a nicer apartment," and finally, in the next to last one, she's saying, "I tell myself I would be a happier person if I were married." And then in the last one, she says, "And then I remember I *am* married."

Whether I was married or not, with or without Sherm going out for the burgers or the ice cream, I would have had my problem with weight. For years, I tried to solve the problem with one fad diet after another. Then, after six years of marriage, I got the good news: I was pregnant.

We were both thrilled. The baby became the focal point of our lives. I was going to be the perfect mother. I would get plenty of rest. I gave up smoking. Exercise, of course, never entered my mind. Or actually, when it did, I pushed the thought away. I really thought it would be dangerous to the baby.

Some women get morning sickness, and I think they're actually the lucky ones. The others, like me, just get hungry. I did eat the proper food most of the time, but I wasn't just eating for two. I was eating for me, the baby, and the Kienast quintuplets.

I started going to my favorite restaurants and having full-course meals. Things like lamb and beans. And that was just lunch. Then I started craving Big Macs. As snacks. Not just one Big Mac. Sacks of Macs. There were so many McDonald's bags in the back of my car that they were a fire hazard. Sherm told me he was considering naming the baby Little Mac.

I didn't look pregnant. I mean, my stomach didn't stick out. What happened was my body started filling out around the stomach. I just looked square. I didn't care. I was in seventh heaven when I discovered maternity clothes: The loose-fitting pants and the big tops were the kind of things I'd been looking for for years.

I didn't want to have to worry about weight. I had deliberately chosen a fat obstetrician. How could she have the nerve to tell me to lose weight? She didn't, and I kept eating, even though the doctor forces you to get on the scales each time you have a prenatal checkup. I couldn't ignore the fact that my weight was soaring.

Well, I'd read all the books about how dangerous it was to get very heavy during pregnancy, and I started to get scared. Up to this point, I hadn't considered myself a binge eater. I considered myself the same as every other woman in America—always dieting to keep from gaining weight. Now I started to feel something was wrong. I was afraid of going off the deep end. Someone recommended that I see a psychiatrist.

The psychiatrist was a man who dealt with addictions—smoking, weight problems, that sort of thing. I can laugh when I look back at this episode in my life, but at the time it wasn't funny. I made an appointment and poured out my story. I didn't leave out a detail—the Big Macs, the lamb, the beans, the works. I did everything but give him the recipes for the stuff I was eating.

When I was finished, this man looked me straight in the eye and told me all these cravings were my way of suppressing my sexual desire. He then went on to tell me that when I got a craving for food, I should try to satisfy the hidden meaning behind that craving. In other words, when I got an urge for two all-beef patties, I should have sex instead. In his opinion, that would solve my problem.

Now folks, my husband worked from 8 A.M. until 5 P.M. and was gone weekends, and I was eating three meals a day plus at least two Big Macs. I also had cravings for food while driving my car, sitting in movies, and strolling through the supermarket. I got so depressed driving home from the doctor's office that I stopped at a McDonald's on the way—this is the truth. I actually went back to see the doctor a second time, because I thought maybe in my pregnant state I had hallucinated the whole thing, but when he gave me the same advice again, I never went back. I think the authorities shut down his operation about a year later.

Meanwhile, I was still eating. I grew out of my maternity clothes. I sat around in my muumuu telephoning friends and trying to get their sympathy.

The nine months went by. Finally, early one morning, my water broke. I was thrilled. I waddled to the car, dashed to the hospital, and checked in. The first thing they did was weigh me. The little mother-to-be weighed 193 pounds.

I was already dilated to three centimeters when the doctor came in to check my stomach. This part is hard to believe, but it's true: She couldn't find the baby.

Needless to say, this made me a little nervous. The doctor was pushing and I was thinking, My God! You mean to tell me I'm not pregnant? Fortunately, a trip to the X-ray department confirmed that indeed a baby was in there. He'd pulled himself into a little ball and scrunched himself all up on one side, probably to make room for all those Big Macs. I'm laughing hysterically as I write this, but it wasn't funny at the time.

Andrew Strelow Pinkham was born six hours later. He weighed a little under six pounds. His mother weighed 193. Yes, folks. I was the first woman in history who didn't lose weight after the delivery. Now, I know there will be a lot of doctors writing to me and telling me this is medically impossible, so I'm going to say that maybe there was some discrepancy between the scale in the check-in and the scale in the maternity ward, but I can tell you whatever it was, the situation didn't do much to lift my postpartum depression.

I was in the hospital for seven days, the oldest mother on the floor. I was twenty-nine. In those days, that was ancient. Since I was in an older and probably more weakened state, I figured it was even more important for me than it was for the other mothers to get my strength back. How? By eating, of course. Besides, I thought eating might cure my post-baby blues, which were severe. I didn't even want visitors.

I told my friends, "No flowers. Just contributions." I asked them to send food. I ate everything in those fruit baskets except the shredded cellophane. I even ate the hospital food, that's how depressed I was. Cream soup that looked and smelled like wallpaper paste. Scrambled eggs you could sip through a straw. Ice cream that made noise when you bit into it.

By the time I was ready to go back home, I had started nursing. I was told that could be my saving grace. Not only was it wonderful for the baby, but it would help me lose weight and tone up. The pregnancy and weight gain had made me pretty buxom, and I was concerned at every feeding that I might smother my child. I stopped nursing Andrew at three months, and it was the first time the child realized you could see and eat at the same time.

Now that Andrew had his good start in life, it was time for me to begin a new diet. I stocked up on all my favorite diet foods— T-bone steak, pork chops, eggs, butter, blue cheese dressing, and a few vegetables that were low in carbohydrates. Dr. Atkins, you almost killed me. I bought your whole premise and with it, half the supermarket's meat and dairy products. I considered those foods— high in calories, high in cholesterol—miracle foods.

I stuck with the diet for a while. Then I started caving in. First I only dreamed about bread. Then I started cheating. An occasional apple. A banana here. A banana there. Still, I was losing weight.

Of course, now I realize that it wasn't what I was or wasn't eating that was causing my weight loss. I was losing weight because I was on the go twenty-four hours a day for the first time in years. Late-night feedings, early-morning feedings, trips to the store, strolls in the park, changing diapers, doing laundry—I was running in circles. But I hadn't put two and two together yet. I thought it was the miracle diet food that was doing the trick. I went down to 160.

Of course, my body wasn't exactly the same. I have a word for those gals who are pregnant. You've got to get that excess baggage off right after the baby's born. Strange things happen to your stomach and your breasts. They never fall exactly back into place again. Then, of course, age itself plays some nasty tricks. Maybe it's not age, exactly, but gravity—gravity and dieting. When you're gaining and losing over and over, something is going to happen to your body, as it did to mine. The cycle was becoming harder to get out of.

I decided to return to work, and after one week on the job I was starting to gain. I was back in the familiar routine. Coffee at home, drive to work, sit four hours, eat lunch, sit some more, drive home, eat dinner, and watch TV. I barely moved. If I had lost the use of my legs, it might have taken me a week or so to discover it.

I was now an addicted dieter. A day wouldn't go by when I wasn't dieting or thinking about dieting. I kept going from 160 to 193 pounds, at least ten times in the past seven years. My body was a mess. I was all flab. It didn't seem to make any difference what the scale read. I was beginning to look the same at any weight—bloated and flabby. Years before, even at 160, I was looking pretty good. Now, at the same weight, I felt mushy. My body had the tone of a water bed. Dieting had destroyed it.

Chapter 4

Success Went to My Waistline

The only fat host you've ever seen on television was Alfred Hitchcock, and if you remember, he dealt in the bizarre. He and I were two rare exceptions on the tube, where everybody from the quiz show contestants to the soap opera stars is in great shape—physically, anyway.

I started appearing on television to promote my book, *Mary Ellen's Best of Helpful Hints*. It was published by Warner Books in 1979, and like most authors, I came to my publisher's offices to discuss publicity. The publicity staff asked me to do a personal appearance tour.

I made my television debut on "Good Morning, Houston." For the occasion, I was wearing a pair of blue polyester pants and a loose smock, which would become my uniform. I thought it made me look like a typical housewife, which it probably did, and I also thought it made me look thinner, which it definitely did not. I did not know either of these things then, or for quite a time afterward, because I would rather have had major dental work without Novocain than look at myself on videotape.

At this point in my life, I hadn't seen any pictures of myself for several years. Frank Sinatra didn't avoid photographers any more diligently than I did, and what few snapshots of me existed, I managed to destroy. I was like a member of some primitive tribe who was afraid the photo would capture his soul, but all I was afraid of was that it would capture the roll around my middle. The only still photos of me that exist were taken before I got married.

There are film archives, though. Sherm bought a movie camera to take pictures after Andrew was born and I didn't have the time to splice myself out of all that film. Besides, I figured that if I did, Andrew wouldn't have any pictures at all of himself and his mom. I left the film alone, but when Sherm showed the movies, I always kept my eyes closed at the scary parts—when I was onscreen.

By the time I started my publicity tour, I weighed about 165. That wasn't the worst I'd been, and it certainly was not the worst I'd get to. Yet, it was enough to make me very self-conscious. People didn't understand how I never worried about what I would *say* on television. Frankly, I was only concerned about my appearance. I always spent much more time preparing for how I was going to look than how I was going to respond to the interviewer. I always knew that my mouth would work, but I didn't know about my face or my body.

That's why I love doing radio. You can have fun and talk and laugh and *nobody can see you.* The first week I was on the road, starting in Houston, I was petrified. Every night I went to bed and I thought, My God, tomorrow I have to get up again and go back on television. The idea was not just frightening, it was awesome.

I think it's interesting that none of my friends ever said anything to me about being fat. Nobody ever sat me down and said, "Mary Ellen, you've got a problem and it's out of control." Before then, the conversations would go, "Mary Ellen, you're such a pretty girl. It would be wonderful if you could take some weight off." Now my appearance was at the point where no one ever brought the subject up, because I wasn't looking pretty at all.

I looked twenty years older. When I was younger, I was complimented on my eyes constantly. But even those comments stopped, because my cheeks had gotten so heavy that my eyes started to look very small. My second chin grew a second chin. "You look a lot like Elizabeth Taylor," one hairdresser told me. "She has no neck either."

When you're fat, you see a fat person on the street and you turn to your friend and say, "Am I as fat as she is?" If you're with a good friend, generally he or she will want to protect you and tell you you're not, even if you actually are.

The only one who said anything to me about losing weight was a stranger who came up to me in the rug department of a Minneapolis department store to tell me the rug I was looking at was overpriced and also I should go on a diet. She was involved in a dieters' group and it had become a religious experience for her: She was a born-again skinny-Minnie. Now I must admit I resented that. One of the worst nuisances about being overweight is that strangers seem to

feel it's an invitation to come up and comment on your appearance—
"You know, you ought to lose some weight"—as if that's something
that never occurred to you. Even if you've avoided mirrors the way I
did, every once in a while you turn a corner and sneak up on
yourself.

Strangers should keep out of it, but I do think good friends
should be able to help you without offending you. At the end of my
fattest period, before I went on the Help Yourself diet, I had become
very demanding and irritable, I was putting myself down constantly, and I was becoming unbearable to be around.

The Mary Ellen everyone knew was disappearing beneath
layers of fat. How did I know? People told me—but not until *after* I'd
begun to lose the weight. I feel that I'm fortunate that I finally
started to diet, but I'm sorry no one felt comfortable helping me face
the facts.

I don't think it helps any fat person if, out of the blue, somebody
close to her just starts telling her she's fat. I think that could drive a
person right into the refrigerator. But a good friend can find the
right time, and should. I know that people found it hard to talk to
me. Evidently I have a forceful personality, though I think I'm a soft
touch and a pushover, and nobody ever had the courage to sit me
down and say gently, "Hey, Mary Ellen, you've got to do something.
You look terrible. You're getting bigger by the month."

And I sure was. I went from being an overweight woman to
being an obese woman. The more successful I became, the more my
eating got out of control. Now, what you usually hear is that the
happier you are, the less likely you'll be fat, because you overeat
when you're sad. Yes, I do eat when I'm sad, but I also eat when I'm
happy. I eat when I'm bored. I eat when food looks good. And I eat a
lot when I'm under stress.

I had felt much more in control of my eating when I was home
all day long. I never really succeeded in my struggle to lose weight,
but I was always diet-conscious. I skipped breakfast and ate a light
lunch, like salad or tuna fish. Dinner was a problem, though. It
usually started around the time the nightly news came on TV and
wrapped up when Johnny Carson and Ed McMahon were saying
good night. On weekends, I looked for a party, and to me partying
meant eating and drinking.

Once *Mary Ellen's Best of Helpful Hints* was published, I was
on the road a lot. I lived in beautiful hotels, and I won't say that

wasn't nice, but I had to deal with the strain of living out of a suitcase and under pressure. I felt a lot of stress. My lifestyle had changed overnight. First, I rationalized: Mary Ellen, in your line of work it isn't important to be thin. I thought that the American housewife could identify with me since I was overweight. I told myself I had a nice home, a good husband, a beautiful child, and a successful career. Maybe, I told myself, you can't expect to have all that *and* a nice trim body.

Of course, one look at Jane Fonda and I should have realized none of that made any sense, but I really believed it. I didn't have much time for self-searching, anyway, on that first tour. I went to twenty cities. A twenty-city tour means you are in an airplane every day and in a new city every night. You work straight through from Monday to Friday, then you go home, and start again on Sunday.

On the road Mondays and Tuesdays, I drank Perrier water and ate salads, with meat and vegetables in the evening. By Thursday at the latest I was out of control. Certainly part of the reason was that I was lonely.

Television seems to be very glamorous. In reality, you walk into the station about half an hour before you go on the air, go to makeup, do the show, pack up your gear, and leave. You don't spend time socially with the people you're talking to on camera for the simple reason that you have to be on a plane that night and on your way, and they have their own lives to lead. It's all quite impersonal. That's not the fault of the people who host the shows, it's just a fact of life.

After the show, you're alone with your thoughts. There is nobody to give you any feedback on your appearance. How did I look? Did I perform well? What could I do to improve myself? Nobody's there to give you reassurance or provide any kind of companionship when you're on the road alone. Food becomes your friend. You look forward to getting into your room, taking a bath, sitting down and having a meal with your pals—protein, fats, and carbohydrates. The meal becomes the high point that you work toward the whole day. Many people admit that they have had the same experience on tour.

A very famous novelist told me that she was midway through a long series of appearances and feeling terrible about the amount of weight she was gaining. One night, just after she had called room service and asked for a big meal, she thought to herself, What am I doing? I don't need all that food, and none of it is any good for me anyway.

So she called down to room service, identified herself, and asked that her order be canceled. The reply she got confirmed all her worst feelings about what she was going to eat: "Sorry, ma'am, we've already put it in the grease."

I have my own favorite depressing room service story. I ordered a fish dinner, and then I changed my mind and told them to forget about the fish and send up a steak instead. (In those days, I didn't realize that fish has fewer calories than steak.)

Whoever took the order must have gotten a little confused, because when I opened the door for room service a little while later, there were two little vases of flowers, two napkins, two sets of silver, and two dinners on the rolling cart. Do you think I sent one back? Not on your life. Waste not, want not, I figured—it was meant to be, and who'll know?

I called out as if someone were in the bathroom. "Hurry up, Katie, your steak is getting cold," and for good measure, "it's just the way you like it." Then I tipped the waiter, let him out the door, and sat down and ate both meals. I even changed seats when I ate the second one.

Eventually, I saw how I looked on television. This happened when I began doing three segments a week for "Good Morning, America." Some were videotaped from my house in Minneapolis. The truck would roll up and the crew would tape and edit on the spot. I didn't want to look like a complete idiot, so I would sit down and watch while they worked.

To my surprise, I didn't look bad. I came to realize this was because when they taped me in Minneapolis, I was onscreen by myself. I always looked okay alone. But the minute you put me next to a normal-sized person, I looked fat. If I were standing next to a TV host, for example, you would notice that his arms were hanging straight down and mine weren't. My hips pushed them out at an angle. It's a look that comes naturally to penguins.

(One host I particularly didn't like standing next to was John Davidson. He's very thin. I secretly considered driving John crazy by paying someone to sneak into his wardrobe closet to take in an eighth of an inch in all his inseams so he'd think he was gaining weight.)

Obviously, I preferred to be sitting if I wasn't alone on camera. I developed a hint for overweight celebrities. One thing about talk shows, and this rule applies from coast to coast, is that they always have one white host, one black host, and a beige couch. What you do is dress in beige. I mean *entirely* in beige—beige suit, beige dress, beige stockings, beige shoes. That way no one knows where you stop and the couch begins.

Someone said she read this in *Cosmopolitan*, but I've been using it at parties for years. I'd call the hostess up and ask what color her sofa was, then dress to match it and get there early enough to plunk down on it. Standing-up parties have never been my favorite for this reason. It's hard to dress to match the wall, particularly if there's wallpaper.

I can admit it now. Underneath those yards of beige, my body was growing fatter and fatter. I was totally out of control. I actually became unconcerned about weight. I decided, "Look, this is the way you are, and this is the way you're going to stay. Accept it. Go forth. Go forth and hint. Go forth and hint and eat."

Sandy Hill from "Good Morning, America" had said to me, when I appeared on the show in the early stages, "What usually happens when people become successful is that they take off the excess weight. You will. I know you will." Of course, eventually, she was right.

But I don't want you to think you need to be successful to get yourself to Help Yourself. In fact, you need it the most when you're feeling down. I have a friend who always plunges into her exercises and is especially careful about what she's eating the minute that life threatens to overwhelm her—the dishwasher has broken down, the kids are driving her crazy, her husband has decided to quit his job as a CPA and become a stand-up comic. She says, "At least I'll have a good body to look forward to."

When you're fat, you're not happy. My book was doing well and I was making good money. For the first time in my life, I could even afford to go to a spa. You know what? I was embarrassed to go. I felt there was no spa that would want me.

I was fat before I had the success with my book and I stayed fat after it took off. The only difference was now I could afford to shop in more expensive fat women's stores.

Chapter 5

Facing the Fat Facts

January 1982. It had been five years since I stepped on a scale. How time flies. The only gauge I had of how serious my weight problem was was the way my clothes fit. Most of them didn't. I was even growing out of my clothes for the larger woman.

At one point, I'd solved the problem of dressing. I had about twenty-five pairs of black slacks. I'd find a brand that was wonderful—in other words, that fit—and I'd buy five at a time. Then I'd put these together with a blouse with long sleeves and a high collar and a black blazer. Dress it up, dress it down. I was set for every occasion. For a funeral, I'd wear the outfit with a gray man-tailored shirt. For a wedding, I'd have a lacy white blouse under the blazer.

This system helped develop my hinting career, because I had a lot invested in preserving my black pants. I figured out creative solutions for every crisis: when they started pulling, when they needed reinforcement at the seams. Finally, when I nearly passed out in my black polyester slacks on one particularly hot July day, I decided I'd had enough.

Then I started going to stores that didn't use standard sizes on the clothes. They were marked A, B, C, and D, or 1, 2, 3, and 4. When the zipper doesn't close on a size D, it's not the same as if it doesn't close on a size 20½. I preferred poking my head out of the dressing room to ask if the same blouse came in a size 4 instead of a 42. If it said "One size fits all" and it didn't, I'd decide the garment was manufactured in one of those countries where the people aren't as large as Americans.

I read in *Vogue* that you don't gain weight in your feet. The people at *Vogue* are obviously not acquainted with serious weight gain. Believe me: Even my feet got fat. I wore a size 6 when I was in high school, and I'd gone up to an 8½. I blamed this on the manufacturers, but I couldn't help noticing that other parts of me were getting fat, unusual parts: fingers and earlobes. My friend looped her thumb and index finger around her wrist to see if she was gaining weight. Not only couldn't I get my thumb and finger to meet, but I also didn't like looking at my wrists. I thought I saw the beginning of stretch marks on them.

Andrew and I had gone to see a revival of Walt Disney's *Cinderella*. Every kid wants to fantasize that he has the most beautiful mother in the world, so when we came out of the movie, I waited expectantly when Andrew asked, "Ma, guess who you remind me of in that movie."

"Who, Andrew?"

"You remind me of that fat little mouse that laughed a lot." Andrew immediately realized he'd hurt my feelings, because he tried to turn his comment into a compliment. I almost wished he had said I reminded him of the wicked stepmother. At least she was thin.

Once again, I vowed I had to do something. The first step would be to confront my body, at this point a stranger to me. I had taken to undressing in the dark. If somehow my head and body got separated, I didn't think I could have picked my body out of a lineup.

There was a time when I used to love to look at my reflection in store windows, but now I didn't even have a full-length mirror in my house. The only mirror I used was on my dressing table, and it was a small one, so I could only see myself from the lips up.

When you get really fat, things you think about a lot are your face and your eye makeup and your hair, not your body. It doesn't exist. Then all of a sudden one day you find yourself walking down the street and you see a fat woman walking toward you and you realize you're walking toward a mirror. Some sane part of me knew I had to see myself as I really looked. Not only did I not want to confront the mirror, but I also knew that once I did I'd convince myself that the mirror was exaggerating the situation.

I started thinking about how when I appeared on television, I'd ask the hosts to give me the "thin camera" and they'd always say "Are you kidding? I keep that one on me." But, of course, the camera doesn't lie. A photograph is incriminating evidence. I decided I should have someone come over and take pictures of me.

The morning the photographer came, I was in a good mood. I decided it would be a fun and games day. I went upstairs and stepped into my maternity pants. Yup, I was still wearing them. I kept them to wear when I was the fattest, and by this time they were really comfortable because they were good and stretched out. I put on a blouse and I tucked it in. Of course, fat people never wear anything tucked in, except maybe a napkin, so that was a sign I really meant business.

On television, I'd learned something about how to pose for pictures. Most heavy people do. Keeping your chin up has real meaning for fat people posing for the camera. They also try to keep their arms up—anything to counter the effects of gravity. Hanging from a trapeze would be good. The major thing is never to face the camera square on; always be photographed in a three-quarters shot. Well, I decided I would do this right, so I really did face the camera. Side *and* front, back and front, sitting on a chair, skirt in, low heels. You've seen those before and after shots in every magazine. The gal looks like a real frump in the before shots—no makeup, messy hair, and no smile. I did some like that, and I also did some in full makeup. I had a really good time, even posing for some gag shots stuffing food in my face.

When the photographs were developed, I can't explain how I felt. I couldn't believe that I had been walking the streets looking like that and no one had made a citizen's arrest: I was defacing the landscape. It was absolutely mindboggling. I couldn't delude myself that it had been a bad day, because in the photos I'd taken in full makeup I looked about as good as I could look.

Normally I would have headed right for the refrigerator, but with the image of those photos in mind, I was too depressed even to do that. There's not a doctor on earth who could have told me to lose weight and convinced me to do it, but these photos did the trick.

I looked back at my dieting history. So far, nothing had worked. What could I do differently this time?

Most diet books tell you to have a physical examination before you go on a diet. Physical examination means you get on a scale, of course. The one at home was gathering dust. I had had a couple of checkups after Andrew was born, but I'd always tell the doctor not to tell me what I weighed. One of the things I'd rather have done than weigh myself was go to war. I truly believe I would rather have died of some disease than get on a scale. I was that obsessed.

But I happened to talk to a gal who told me that she'd had a major weight problem, and the doctor had discovered it was all because she had an underactive thyroid. He'd given her some pills and bingo! She lost forty pounds. Well, of course I thought this was sensational news. I was thoroughly convinced I had a thyroid problem. All I had to do was go to the doctor and get the thyroid pills and I'd be Miss America in six months.

I made an appointment.

The day before I went, I didn't eat. The night before I went, I didn't sleep. I took a laxative. If I'd had some diuretics, I'd have taken a few of those. I was hoping the doctor wouldn't absolutely have to weigh me, but I knew it wasn't likely. Even the dermatologists weigh you. I used to say I'm here for my skin, not my waist, but those nurses would get me on the scale before I knew what was happening. When I got to this doctor, it was clear the nurse meant business, too.

Of course, I don't think a nurse's task is an easy one. If I were a nurse, I'd see to it that all fat patients were sedated before they weighed in. I'm probably typical. First I gave her a hard time about my height. When I was in high school, I considered myself a medium-boned woman of average height, but the fatter I got, the more I liked to think of myself as large-boned and tall. The nurse had the nerve to tell me I was only five foot five. I indicated that I had my doubts about her competence.

She had her revenge, of course, by weighing me. She just kept moving those counterweights to the right. Finally, she got the scales to balance. What was very amazing to me was that lights didn't go off, bands didn't march in, and no "tilt" signs started flashing. No one fainted. I *nearly* did. I weighed 208 pounds. What helped me keep my composure was that the nurse who was weighing me looked as if she were good for about 250 pounds herself.

Okay, so that was the news. I was more than seventy pounds overweight. Even so, just by going to the doctor's office and facing the scale, I felt as though a big burden had been taken off my shoulders. It was still around my stomach, of course. But being in the doctor's office was just another sign to me that I meant business, that I'd just taken another big step. Who really cared what the nurse thought? Being there was a signal to me that I had some self-esteem left.

I hadn't met the doctor at this point. The doctors never weigh you in, of course. They give all the dirty work to nurses. Eventually he walked in, washed his hands, and then gave me his full attention.

"Well, well, well," he said. "What do we have here?"

They always say that. "Well, well, well. What do we have here?" At 208 pounds, it was awfully hard to miss what he had there. I told him what I thought he had: a person with a weight problem who needed her blood pressure checked. A person who, I advised him, probably had a thyroid problem.

The doctor took a few tests and called me back to his office. The tests had all come back negative. I was in good health. The doctor said, specifically, "You are in good health." I was never so disappointed in my life. "You are in good health," he repeated, peering over his glasses, "but you are fat." I hoped he wasn't charging me a lot for this diagnosis.

My blood pressure was a bit high, he said, and my heart rate was, too, but he felt they would come down if I lost some weight.

What I really wanted was a thyroid pill. I was convinced that my thyroid was a mess. It's not as if I hadn't made several serious stabs at losing weight. Even if I cut back drastically, I told the doctor, I didn't lose weight. Amazingly, as I look back, I realize that he never asked if I exercised. He just handed me a 1500-calorie-a-day diet and gave me a lecture telling me to stick to it. In other words, he had no real solution for me.

My worst moment was when my glance fell on my folder lying open on his desk. It said "obese." "Obese" is a word that even if you don't know the language you would stay away from. It's not a word I've ever been fond of, particularly as applied to myself. I was devastated. I would rather have served a prison sentence than be called "obese."

Before I got through the front door of the office, I started rationalizing. I had been through a rough experience, so I needed food. I drove out of the doctor's parking lot and into the restaurant's next door. I ordered a salad and diet soda, which I suppose meant something—I could have asked for a burger, fries, and a Coke—but the point is that I was still using food as a crutch. When I faced a problem, it was the first thing I thought of.

I was very desperate. I started thinking about a stomach stapling or intestinal bypass. I can't tell you exactly how they're done, but surgically the doctor fixes up your insides so you don't keep enough food in your system to gain weight. It sounded good to me. I called various doctors in the area requesting either process, but I was told you had to be at least a hundred pounds overweight to be considered for the procedure. I wasn't quite one hundred pounds overweight, so for one brief moment I considered eating my way up to qualify. Fortunately, before I began working my way through Minneapolis' McDonald's franchises, I read something pretty horrifying: Stomach staples pop and bypasses become ineffective. Somehow, within two years of the operation, most patients gain the weight back. Plus, thanks to whatever the doctors have done to your insides, you put in quite a few hours in the ladies' room, if you know what I mean. That put me off. In fact, this was one of the reasons I'd never tried the Beverly Hills diet, which is heavy on roughage. I can think of nicer ways to spend my free time.

So I did the only thing I knew how to do. I started to crash diet. I deprived myself completely. I ate almost nothing all day, slept about ten hours, and barely moved. I was like a dry alcoholic who has given up drinking but continues to show the same obnoxious personality traits. They're belligerent and demanding. They think, I'm a good guy, you're a bad guy, I'm deprived, I'm not drinking, the world owes me something. They haven't changed their attitude about living. The only difference is they're not sitting around with a glass of Old Forester in their hands.

That's how I was acting. I felt deprived. I felt angry. Why me, God? I thought. Why should I weigh 208 pounds? I'm a great person. What have I done to deserve this? And the more you think like this, the more you want to eat. Alcoholics have the same experience, only they want to drink.

The longer this went on, the more I was convinced that something was truly wrong, and I was determined to do something about it. I had to find a diet that I could live with. I didn't know what it would be, but I knew I couldn't go back to doing anything I had done in the past. My first thought was to fast, to check into a hospital and live on liquid protein; but I had done similar things in the past and I knew they didn't work.

Remember Scarlett O'Hara out in her garden, looking at the sky and vowing she'd never go hungry again? Well, I went outside to my garden and vowed I'd never be hungry and fat at the same time again. There had to be some explanation for what was going wrong with my body, and I decided if it took me until the day I died, I was going to find out what it was and get the fat off in the process.

It made me feel better to have made this decision, but I had to find somebody who'd help me find the answers.

Thank goodness, I got the flu.

Chapter 6

What's Up, Doc?

After my experience with Dr. 1500-Calories-a-Day, I made a vow to stay away from anyone dressed in white unless he sold ice cream. Then I came down with the flu. For a while I was in heaven—after all, I was losing weight.

After a few days, my friends and loved ones advised me that my coughing and wheezing and whooping and monopolizing of the john were rapidly becoming a pain in the neck. Besides, I had a very important business meeting coming up. One of the fellows I worked with insisted I should see his physician, Dr. Joel Holger.

I like my doctors a little overweight with gray hair. Dr. Joel was blond and looked exactly like a ski instructor, minus the parka. That, combined with the fact that he seemed unusually nice, led me to wonder if he was a bona fide doctor, but he had the right certificates hanging up in his office, the pharmacy honored his prescription without any question, and he cured my flu, so I guessed he was.

I actually liked him. Every once in a while we'd run into each other socially, and it got to the point where I'd drop by his office so we could have coffee and talk a little, which for me is the equivalent of Red Riding Hood paying a social call on the wolf. I kept expecting him to give me what I thought of as "the doctor lecture" about my weight, but he never made it an issue. I even tested him. If we were out and everyone was having pizza, I'd take a slice just to see if he'd say, "Put that down, Mary Ellen, you're ready to explode," but he never did. The truth is that I'd already made a commitment to myself and was attempting to control my weight. I wasn't gaining—but I wasn't losing, either. Dr. Joel was aware of this because I'd mentioned it in passing, but we didn't discuss it right away. Then, little by little, I started expressing my concern.

I discovered that Dr. Joel, who specializes in internal medicine, was very interested in nutrition, and from time to time he'd mention some fact passed on by friends who were doing research in the field.

He told me that there were a lot of new discoveries about weight control that might be important and helpful to me, and finally he suggested that maybe we should get together and talk about it sometime. I agreed. For one thing, I trusted him. For another, I had run out of diets. I was eating very little most days, and the weight wasn't coming off.

The day we had our first discussion I was sitting on Dr. Joel's couch. Actually, I was sitting on part of his couch. In those days, at my fattest, I always removed the back cushion on sofas. That left more room for my body.

Once I was nice and comfortable, we decided to start at the beginning. Dr. Joel asked me to describe the diets I'd gone on in chronological order. I was really proud as the minutes passed by. I calculated I'd been on over seventy diets. Dr. Joel had already developed writer's cramp by the time I was up to 1971.

"Sorry," he said when we were finished. "I have to tell you you're an addict—a diet addict." Of course, he said, I wasn't the only one. The majority of American women are addicted dieters.

I knew that. Dieting isn't just a means to an end anymore, it's the fashion. If you're dieting, that means you care about how you look. If you're not dieting, you're a schlep. Even the kids know this. My friend's little three-year-old son refused to wear a white suit she'd bought him. Why? He came up with the excuse he'd heard from the grownups: "It makes me feel fat." My own son Andrew, who hasn't got an ounce to spare anywhere on his body, sometimes asks, "Ma, when can I go on a diet?"

Today, right after they say, "How are you?" people don't ask "What's new?" or "How're things?" like they used to. They say, "You're looking thin," which means good. I do it myself. I did a guest appearance on a show with Orson Welles once and I told him *he* looked thin.

"How are you?" means hello. "Have a good day" is a form of saying good-bye. When people say it, I usually want to jump off a balcony, but they say it anyway. The whole rest of the conversation gets squeezed in between "How are you? You're looking thin" and "Have a good day." Only when you're walking away do they turn to a friend and say, "Boy, she's looking fat."

And of course I was, which is the reason I'd finally come to Dr. Joel. After he took my history, he really endeared himself to me by not weighing me right away. First, he spent some time explaining why every one of the fad diets I went on was a nutritional disaster. "You're kidding," was my first reaction. "Even that nice lady who tells me to stuff my face with pineapple is talking through her hat?" On top of that, he told me that there is no food that burns fat. Was I disappointed! I felt like the kid who learned that there is no Easter Bunny and no Santa Claus. On the same night.

Worse news. A lot of these diets are truly dangerous. Calories-don't-count diets—the ones that are low in carbohydrates and high in fat—strain your kidneys. Others are lacking in bulk, or Vitamin C, Vitamin A, or potassium. Really strict diets, especially when they lack protein, are very dangerous. If you don't take in enough food to meet your body's energy requirements, the body breaks down its own tissue—even tissue from vital organs like your heart. (What's the difference between a vulture and a fad diet? The vulture waits until you're dead before it eats your heart out.)

As fast as I could come up with some other diet I'd been on, Dr. Joel would tell me how it could kill me. Still, that wasn't the worst news he delivered about dieting, and if you're a fat person, you'll know what I mean.

The worst news was that *dieting helps make you fat.*

Dr. Joel explained it all scientifically, but I have to confess I missed most of what he was saying the first time around. All I could think of was that nobody had told me the truth. All those ladies' magazines and all those diet books I'd read, and all those doctors I'd seen talking to Merv and Johnny and Mike weren't really giving me the whole story. I never believed everything I read in the papers or all the claims in the commercials, but I believed everybody who came out with a new miracle diet. Now it turned out that I shouldn't have. No fad diet helped me do anything but get fatter.

It seems that there are two main causes for what Dr. Joel insisted on calling "obesity." I told him that was one of my least favorite words, but he said that "overweight" was—for reasons he'd soon explain—not really accurate.

One reason is primary hyperphagia, which in plain English means overeating. The other is primary obesity, which in simple terms is a tendency to get fat. We primary obesity types, the scientists now think, may react to long-term rigid dieting by increasing our fat production.

This made sense to me. Sure, I overeat some things. Who doesn't? Even the thinnest people I know sometimes eat dessert when they're not really hungry for it. But it seemed as if I were cutting down on my food over the years and still getting fatter and fatter. It wasn't just a lack of willpower that kept me fat, Dr. Joel was saying, it was actually the diets I went on.

There seems to be some evidence that every one of us has what authors William Bennett, M.D., and Joel Gurin describe in *The Dieter's Dilemma* as a setpoint—a weight our bodies go to unless we're restricting our calories. That's why some of us are always battling the same ten pounds and why even though others get fat, they don't go all the way up to circus-fat-lady size. In my teens, my setpoint was around 135. My setpoint, in postpregnancy, was 193. No matter how I dieted, I always wound up back there if I stopped watching what I was eating.

Dieting, it turns out, can't lower the setpoint. We fat people have been on diets constantly. And the result of constant dieting is to lower the rate at which you burn food—your basal metabolism.

Dr. Joel explained that the human body is designed for survival. It was designed so we could go for very long periods without food, in the days when there were no twenty-four-hour supermarkets and all-night diners. And the most efficient way to store food, he further explained, is in fat because it's concentrated. Fat has more calories per pound than carbohydrates or protein; for example, a tablespoon of butter (fat) is more fattening than a tablespoon of rice (carbohydrate) or fish (protein).

Our bodies are very clever about saving up the fat stores. When you diet and lower your food intake, your body lowers its fuel-burning rate so the food will burn more slowly. Your body thinks, we must be stranded on a desert island somewhere. Less food is coming in. So we'd better burn our supplies more slowly. And this happens even if your body has plenty of fat already tucked away for an emergency. It's as if your body has landed on a desert island but doesn't realize that the *Queen Elizabeth* is washed up alongside it.

Anyway, pretty soon you stop dieting, and you're off the island and back into McDonald's. Your body doesn't know this right away (news is slow to travel from the mainland), so it continues to burn food more slowly.

You're taking in the same amount of food as you did before you began dieting, but your body is burning that food more slowly. You're gaining weight. If you happen to be taking in a little extra, in a postdiet splurge, you not only gain back what you lose, but a few extra pounds besides. How long your basal metabolism rate is set off-kilter is not certain—but it is long enough to permit a weight gain.

As if that weren't bad enough, the new, heavier you is composed of a higher proportion of fat than when your diet began. If you lose twenty pounds, ten is probably water, five lean muscle, and five fat. What you regain is ten pounds of water and ten of fat, assuming you don't exercise.

The more muscle there is in your body, the faster you burn calories, even at rest, just in the simple acts of breathing and circulating blood. On the other hand, fat tissue uses up calories much more slowly. The new, fatter you needs even less calories than before you dieted, but you probably haven't cut your usual caloric intake, have you? This is a second reason for weight gain.

I was a textbook case. My metabolism had gone haywire, my body composition was too high in fat, and with each new diet I was struggling harder to lose weight. The worst part of it was that my setpoint, which had been around 135, had moved up to 193 and, like inflation, seemed to be going higher with no end in sight.

Could I move it back down?

Could I get my metabolism operating like a normal person's?

Could Mary Ellen Pinkham, a gal from the Midwest, find happiness as a thin person?

Yes. Dr. Joel finally delivered a piece of good news. He told me that all the evidence seemed to indicate that you can improve your metabolic rate. He had a theory about it, and he asked me if I'd like to be a guinea pig (which I suggested wasn't the most tactful phrase). A test case? What the heck, I told him. I'd done whatever every crackpot who wore a stethoscope told me to do and followed the advice of a few crackpots without them. Now, someone I trusted wanted me to try his method. How could I refuse? I had nothing to lose but my weight.

Part of his theory involved reducing my caloric intake. A diet, in other words. But there was a new twist. Over the course of the diet, as I lost weight, Dr. Joel would slowly add to my daily calories. He was certain that his system would permit me to ultimately take in hundreds of calories a day more than I was now eating and stabilize at a normal weight. To break the crash and binge syndrome, it was important that I get my metabolism used to a normally high intake.

I had been either dieting or gaining weight for as long as I could remember. There was no in-between for me. And none of the fad diets I'd ever been on ever paid much attention to what happened once the diet was over. The idea that I could, at some point, eat like a normal person was very appealing.

A nutritionist would work out the details of the diet, and Dr. Joel thought I should help her set the ground rules. I also wanted a very strict plan. Nutritionists think structured diets are a bad idea. They say that people want to "rebel" against them, and structured diets don't teach you how to select food for yourself. But I wasn't ready to make my own choices. For one thing, I really didn't know much about caloric values. Besides, we addicted dieters are so used to rigid rules that we need and like them. Our past dieting history has turned us into robots. Tell us what to eat, how much, what time, and we'll do it. We're incapable of making choices because we're afraid of making the wrong ones, and if we do, the miracle—fast weight loss—won't happen. Dr. Joel and I compromised: I would start with a strict plan, then go on an unstructured one once I felt capable of taking control.

I also thought the nutritionist should give me a shopping list for the strict plan part of the diet, and I asked for other considerations.

1. Keep me out of the supermarket. I only wanted to shop once a week.
2. Keep me out of the kitchen. If I wasn't supposed to spend a lot of time eating, I didn't want to spend a lot of time cooking (and tasting).
3. Don't plan for any leftovers. I am a member of the Clean Plate Club Hall of Fame. I have eaten meals on behalf of the starving peoples of every nation. I am unable to prepare a recipe that serves four and eat only a quarter of it. If a diet calls for half a cantaloupe, I worry about what will become of the other half, so I eat it. But if I know I'm supposed to save it for a meal later in the week, I will.

We agreed that the diet would begin on January 31. I would go to Dr. Joel's office for instructions about the nondiet part of his plan, which he hadn't yet explained to me.

I had long since gotten past the point of postponing diets to Monday mornings. At this point in my life, I planned on going on diets every day. In honor of the occasion, I'd often have a big blowout the night before. My friend LizBeth actually started the tradition of Farewell to Food celebrations. She had refined the system so that she would actually have a theme to her eating. I remember Ebony and Ivory Eve, Mint Monday, and White-on-White Night, which was my favorite. It started with potato soup, and continued with turkey on white bread, followed by rice pudding and sponge cake with French vanilla ice cream, marshmallow topping, and blanched almonds.

Typically, after eating on a Farewell to Food night, I would go to sleep and have a deprivation dream. An ice-cream vendor would refuse to sell me Chipwiches. All the souvlaki stands in New York burned down. Management closed the Reese's factory.

But on January 30, 1982, I dreamed that I was at a party. Gloria Vanderbilt was offering me a tray of hors d'oeuvres, and she was saying, "You're much too thin."

I knew this time would be different.

Chapter 7

The Moving Experience

Dr. Joel was ready for me on January 31. He had even removed the back cushion from his sofa so I could settle in comfortably.

We had worked out the details of the diet. Now he was going to explain the other part of the program. "You're going to exercise," he said.

Exercise? That was the secret weapon he was going to use? Visions appeared before me. Situps. Pushups. Me in a leotard. Richard Simmons ordering me to do one hundred leg-lifts. I told Dr. Joel he had to be kidding.

I was well acquainted with the argument that stepping up physical activity is an ineffective way to lose weight. I remember reading a magazine article about twenty years ago that said in order to burn off a pound of fat, you had to walk from Mexico to California. Or maybe it said you had to walk ten miles. Whatever it was, it seemed a long way to me.

That article cinched it. I thought, What is this? You have to put in that much effort to burn off a pound of fat?

So from the time I was in my teens, I looked for diets that discouraged physical activity. Most of them did. They never actually said exercise was forbidden, but they were always accompanied by little charts that told you you had to cha-cha for ten hours straight and then chop down the Yellowstone National Forest to work off the calories in an apple. I reminded Dr. Joel of all of this.

Then he told me a couple of things. The newest research shows that exercise might be helpful in speeding up your entire fuel-burning mechanism. In other words, scientists now think that when you exercise, you don't only burn up a set number of calories, but also you speed up your rate of burning. And this effect might last for as long as twenty-four hours after you have exercised.

Also, and especially important for someone like me, there is a good chance that exercise can reverse the damage done by dieting. Dr. Joel reminded me that as a result of going on my very first diet, I'd lost muscle. It's harder to break down fat than muscle, so when I cut down my caloric intake, my body went to the most easily available source of extra calories—my lean muscle mass. When I regained weight, I gained fat, because you only regain muscle if you exercise, which I had not done.

That's why Dr. Joel told me I shouldn't think of myself as overweight, but overfat. There are some people who weigh exactly what they should on the charts, but the fat content of their body is too high in proportion to the lean muscle mass. You've seen them, with their little pot bellies and flabby arms. Ideally, women's bodies should be composed of about 22 percent fat. I didn't know what percent fat I was, but I had a suspicion that if I got too near a flame, I'd melt.

Dr. Joel said that by exercising, you can change the proportion of fat and muscle in your body. The larger the proportion of muscle to fat in your body, the more calories your body uses at all times. Muscle uses more calories than fat just to go through the processes of daily life. An athlete in good shape uses more calories to breathe than a thin person does. Standing around, looking good, Chris Evert Lloyd burns up more calories than I did running around the block. It didn't seem fair.

Yet Dr. Joel's explanation made sense to me. In my opinion, I was moving around quite a bit, but my body just wasn't burning the calories properly. What about shopping? I was doing a lot of shopping. Didn't moving around from store to store count for anything? Look how thin Jackie Onassis is. I was shopping all the time and it wasn't doing a thing for my body.

Also, I did walk around the lake once or twice a month. Of course I didn't enjoy it. I dreaded it. Every step I took was agony. I knew it was important to give your body a real workout every once in a while, and I thought my biweekly walks were good for me. As a matter of fact, I figured they were especially good since they hurt. Physical activity in my mind was equated with pain. The theory was, "No pain, no gain."

Dr. Joel asked me to write down as best I could what I had done for the past couple of days. I had just come back from a trip to New York, and I had spent the day before this one going about my regular work routine. I'd spent two very busy days running from appointment to appointment. Well, "running" wasn't exactly accurate. Dr. Joel asked how I got from place to place. Of course I went by cab in New York or by car in Minneapolis. I almost never went on foot. The automobile is the American way. Traveling by car is very patriotic, I told Dr. Joel, since it supports the auto industry.

Dr. Joel said that my heart was in the right place even if it was buried under layers of fat. He suggested that if I really felt the auto industry needed my support, I could make a donation to the Chrysler company. Then he told me an amazing piece of information. He had read that the activity level for Americans had fallen so dramatically that the average person would easily have gained twenty pounds in the last twenty years if he had not also cut down his food intake.

When I thought about that a little, I realized I had seen it happening firsthand in the difference between my mother's generation and my own. I don't remember my mother ever going to exercise class or taking any kind of regular exercise. Yet she and her friends never really had a weight problem, and they all ate three square meals a day. (Plus, I remember a lot of kaffeeklatsches in between meals, with lots of real cream and sugar and homemade pastry on the table.) Why? They were truly physical beings.

We all lived in two- or three-story houses, and that meant a lot of running up and down. And every day had its share of demanding household chores. When our mothers did a wash, they had to hang the clothes on the line to dry and then they had to iron them. When was the last time anyone I knew ironed an hour a day—or an hour a week?

We didn't have wall-to-wall carpeting. We had rugs, and even though we did have vacuums—I'm not that ancient—I remember my grandmother taking the rugs out once a month and throwing them over the clotheslines and beating the heck out of them.

We walked to the stores. You didn't make a weekly trip to the supermarket, you walked to the grocery store whenever you needed things, and you walked to the butcher and the baker and the hardware store. Everybody walked. I had to admit that if I compared that shopping to my couple of spins around the air-conditioned mall, I really wasn't getting much exercise.

It's funny that during my childhood you never saw a grown-up at the lake. Oh, once in a while the other kids and I would spot what we considered a weirdo taking a run, but the lake was mostly just ours. Today, there are bicycle paths, jogging paths, and hiking paths, and a lot of people are on them, but most of us are just kidding ourselves. We take the exercise class once a week, but let's face it: We're sedentary.

Dr. Joel didn't want me to do any exercise other than walking. Somehow, "walking" didn't really seem like "exercise" to me. For "exercise," you need equipment. My usual pattern on the few occasions when I decided I might get some exercise was to outfit myself for it. (A bonus in this plan was that I could put off doing the exercise until I got to the sporting goods store.) Buying the outfits was the only truly pleasurable part of exercising for me. I think that dated back to my teenage years, when I had positive feelings about my high school gym uniform. It had a blue bottom with a white top, and we had our names embroidered on the top. My mother was a great seamstress and she could really embroider. She did my name in very decorative embroidery, and since it was Mary Ellen Higginbotham, it stretched out very nicely across the top of my pocket clear around my back, and really stood out. (Of course, that goes to show how thin I was. In recent years I could have crammed the whole name between my pocket and my underarm.)

I had not only become convinced that exercise was relatively pointless in weight control, but I also was having a harder time finding the clothes in my size, with the possible exception of football jerseys. Besides, I didn't think I cut a really impressive figure. You don't look like a Davis Cup challenger in a size 44 tennis skirt. As for exercise class, the word "tights" has new meaning when they're stretched around thighs that are the same size a waist is supposed to be. My thinking was, I can't show up at exercise class until I lose weight. I'll look better and move better then, and I won't embarrass myself as much. The truth is that a lot of fat people are very agile, but they don't want to expose themselves in public, which is a very sad thing.

At one point, I was going to take up jogging. There was one very attractive feature to jogging that I could see. The clothing has elastic waists. I got myself a nice blue velour outfit and blue shoes and blue socks and a blue knit cap and blue sunglasses. I even got myself a jogging bra, that's how serious I was. I felt terrific. The only thing that didn't work out was the jogging itself. (Fortunately, the outfit wasn't a complete waste. I wore it to a Halloween party and told everyone I'd come as the Pacific Ocean.)

Dr. Joel made it clear he was not telling me to jog. I was supposed to walk. He showed me how to test my pulse to see if my pace was brisk enough. But the most important thing was that I was to do it no less than five times a week and never skip two days in a row. Of course, you don't have to be a doctor to know that going out and playing a couple of exhausting sets of tennis just a couple of times a year wins you the key to Heart Attack City. But it turns out that regular exercise is not only safer, but it also increases the benefit of the exercise. According to the estimates, exercising four or five times a week is three times as effective as exercising only three times a week; and exercise once or twice a week has little effect at all.

Dr. Joel also made me take my measurements. I was in perfect proportion—exactly ten inches too much of me in every key spot. I asked Dr. Joel if by any chance he had any suggestions—since I was going to be exercising anyway—for doing something about my cellulite. You don't have cellulite, he said. So, I figured, maybe I'm being too hard on myself. Maybe my hips are fine. No, Dr. Joel said, there is indeed something on your hips, but it's just fat, in another shape. There is no such thing as cellulite.

And there is no such thing as spot-reducing. (I felt really bad when I thought of the hours I'd wasted walking my hips along the floor. I couldn't say I'd miss doing it, though.)

Dr. Joel pointed out that if spot-reducing really worked, gum chewers wouldn't have double chins and typists would always have skinny fingers. He explained further that if you do a lot of situps, your stomach muscles will be in great shape, but if you're still too fat, they'll be buried under a layer of marshmallow.

It seems that walking exercises the largest sets of muscles in your body, and when you exercise large sets of muscles, fat is drawn from all over your body. My thighs and all the other parts of my body that were too fat would slim down without any exercise other than walking. It sounded too good to be true, but I committed myself to go through with Dr. Joel's plan.

On February 1, I started the diet and exercise program. I knew I'd have more trouble with the exercising than the diet. After all, I'd been on diets before. Of course, I'd never dieted and exercised together. I wouldn't have considered it possible. Everyone knows you need extra food when you exert yourself. Doubling the day's caloric intake for every five minutes of exercise seemed like a good rule of thumb to me in the past.

But I was determined to stick to this program. Dr. Joel had cleverly started me with a pretty modest exercise program. Part of my whole way of life is to think that if a little of something is good, a lot is better. If someone tells me to exercise for five minutes, then I think I should go out and do thirty. Of course, the next day I'm so worn out I don't want to do any. Dr. Joel understood this, so he told me to start by walking twenty minutes, and twenty minutes only.

On February 1, I got up and walked for twenty minutes and then I came back and ate my breakfast. In those twenty minutes, just walking briskly, measuring my pulse rate the way I was supposed to, I actually worked up a little sweat.

The next day I decided to do my twenty minutes at lunchtime, so I drove myself over to the lake and walked around for twenty minutes, then drove myself back to the office.

This went on for a week. I was doing my walking, but it was like taking medicine. I hated it. I never experienced any pain, because a twenty-minute walk just didn't do that, but the twenty minutes seemed like an hour. I was doing it because I had to.

I sat down and took a critical look and realized I was going out of my way to do the walking. In the morning, I forced myself to go ten minutes from my house and then turn around and come back. I wasn't going anywhere, or looking at anything, and I was taking the same path every day. At lunchtime, I drove for two miles to take my little twenty-minute spin. It was ridiculous.

I said to myself, "Mary Ellen, you're the kind of person who needs a purpose to what you're doing. Some people would enjoy walking aimlessly, but you don't. So give yourself a destination." That Sunday I walked to church. I was up to thirty minutes by then, and that got me there. I felt so good that after church was over, I turned around and walked home. I started walking to visit my friends. I started walking to the grocery store.

Then I started looking at my other alternatives. I decided that I could try walking to work. It was exactly the right distance for an hour walk. I treated myself to a cassette player with headsets, got some great tapes, and off I went. I was my own car. And the more I walked myself around, the more I enjoyed it.

Friends who were runners used to tell me they couldn't stand to miss a day. "I've got to get out and run. I don't feel good when I haven't moved," they'd tell me, and I couldn't understand this. The amazing thing was that in a matter of two weeks of exercising every single day, my body started to crave exercise, too.

I can't say there weren't setbacks, but I just kept plugging away. The only thing that was really important was getting out the front door. Once I'd done that, I found I could always keep going. One day I found myself whistling as I walked. For a change, I wasn't feeling sorry for myself; I was actually enjoying the walk. That was the day I really got hooked—and it was only a month into the program.

An added reward that came along was the wonderful times walking gave me with my son. I had been really inactive before and now Andrew started looking forward to going out with me. Before, our activities had always centered around food. Maybe we'd go out to a movie first, but the big treat was always going out for what I euphemistically referred to as "a bite" to eat. My little boy did not like sitting in restaurants. He wanted to be out doing something, and once he found out that I would be going along with him, he said, "Anytime, any day, Mom. You can wake me up early. I'll go with you." He hopped on his bike and rode back and forth while I walked alongside him.

There isn't one thing about the walking that hasn't made me feel good. I've probably moved more since January of this year than I have since I was nineteen. I don't roll out of bed anymore, I spring out. New verbs have entered my life: skip, run. In New York, I used to take cab rides that were so short the meter didn't even jump. Now what's jumping is me. I don't use the excuse that I can't walk because I'm wearing high heels; I keep my tennis shoes in a very nice canvas carryall that I carry everywhere.

I used to take my legs for granted. Now, when I walk, I feel them carry me along. Sometimes I look down and watch them move. I think about how they're getting firmer and stronger with every step. I imagine that with each one, I'm leaving a little bit of fat behind.

And then, midway through the diet, those same legs betrayed me. They took me out for a binge.

Chapter 8

When the Compliments Stop

Picture it. I'm at the halfway point. One hundred and sixty-five pounds. Somewhat less than a Green Bay Packer, quite a bit more than a Russian gymnast, and holding. I haven't lost an ounce in two weeks. Am I mad? Will I get my revenge? Of course. I'll eat something. The only question is what. I'm in New York, an eater's paradise.

I put on a beltless dress and hit the streets, just another New Yorker striding along with a purpose. Mine happens to be cake.

I turn into the first likely spot, one of those places with baked goods on revolving stands in the window. The cakes are very tall, nearly as tall as the hairdo of the hostess who seats me. The waiter hands me the menu and I turn directly to the last page. It's called "The Grand Finale." A whole page of desserts. I go for something simple: a slice of chocolate fudge cake a la mode with a glass of skim milk on the side. What's cake without milk?

The order is there in no time. As the waiter puts it in front of me, he gives me a little smile. "Enjoy, gorgeous," he says.

Yes. He said "gorgeous." I'm saved. I want to jump up and kiss him. I'm not hungry anymore. I leave the cake and milk untouched, put a large tip beside it, pay the check, and go out the door.

Until not too long ago, there was always someone offering a psychological explanation for binging. It was the result of unresolved conflicts in my life or a dieting depression that just overpowered my willpower. Then the American Psychological Association said being fat was a physical problem only—not a psychological one. That pleased me: I never much liked the idea that I was fat because I was some kind of psychological mess.

Of course, in the long run, it didn't matter. I was dieting and exercising to get my metabolism working again, and no matter what caused me to binge, I had to find a way to stop it.

As usual, my first few days on the program had been a breeze. Sure, I was eating less, and walking more, than I wanted to, but the beginning of a diet is like the beginning of a love affair. You feel proud and optimistic, and you have someone to daydream about all the time: your future self.

Within a very few days, between the walking and the dieting, I had lost six pounds. I thought, "Boy, I'm in control. I have several good days behind me." I wanted to speed things up. My urge was to start fasting. I felt like Mother Theresa, full of goodwill toward myself and others, cleansed, and a little fragile, which at 202 pounds is some indication of what a wonderful imagination I have. Dr. Joel reminded me that if I crashed, I wouldn't be taking off fat anyway. Most of what you lose when you crash is just water. He advised me to sit back and relax and follow the program.

But I was on such a high, I was so sure I was in control, that I couldn't wait for a chance to test myself. People were starting to invite me out to dinner. I was still on the first few days of the program, the very restricted part, but I thought, "I can handle this," and off I went.

I found myself with my hand in the breadbasket, then dipping my breadsticks into the butter, and eventually I realized then and there I wasn't ready to be out eating. The evening turned out to be a positive experience, though, because I found I was able to ignore the slip and just start right back on the program. Besides, the diet menus were good and eating three meals a day not only satisfied me, it was a novelty.

Staying on the program became even a little easier as soon as I began to get the compliments from my husband and friends. I loved the attention. It was terrific. All I wanted to talk about was how wonderful I was starting to look, how great I felt, and what I was and wasn't eating. If a conversation wasn't about me, I felt that at least it should be led by me.

My friend Ian invented a little imaginary event he called the Boring Olympics. There were a variety of competitions, such as Speed Boring and Long-Distance Boring. He told me that Mary Ellen and her diet and her walking were taking top honors in all of them. I was becoming the Number One World Class bore.

Enough already, I told myself. Lives are going on, the seasons are changing, Liz is having marital problems, there's a new heir to the throne of England, there are other subjects to talk about than how loose your waistband is. Put things in perspective. People want to talk about more than how you look and your diet program. Enjoy the compliments and shut up.

Then came the really rough period. The compliments did stop. That made it very hard for me. I was working hard to stay on the program, my weight had plateaued so I didn't even get any satisfaction out of stepping on the scale, and my diet and I had lost the Number One spot on the Hot Topic Parade. That's what led me to the cake.

When the waiter helped snap me out of my mood, I realized that I needed a lot of attention to help keep me going. If people keep telling you how great you look, not only does it make you feel good, but you're also a lot less likely to pile extra helpings on your plate.

I made a point of getting out among friends. In the past, when I'd go on a crash diet, often I'd lock myself up, go to bed early, do anything possible to keep myself away from humanity and food. Well, you can hibernate for maybe two weeks if you're a social creature like I am. I knew I'd be on this diet a lot longer than two weeks, so I had to find a way to be social without overindulging.

After my slip at the dinner party, I did limit my activities in the very beginning, but after a couple of weeks, the diet had become part of my routine. Besides, Dr. Joel insisted that I keep a book and write down everything I ate all day, together with the calorie count. This seemed especially silly to me in the beginning, when I was following the diet he gave me exactly, but it was a little like writing out the multiplication tables when you're a kid. By the time I'd written down "1 medium-sized baked potato—100 calories" a few times, I knew the calorie count without thinking. I had a better idea of what damage I'd do if I took a little taste of this and that. I'll never forget the day I was looking through the calorie book and I noticed that Roquefort dressing had 100 calories. Per *tablespoon*. I wanted to call all my friends to warn them. I didn't know where to write to complain.

I had never been one of those people who went to a party for the food rather than the conversation, but I did find it was a good idea if I positioned myself a little farther than usual from the cocktail and buffet tables.

When discussion of my weight wore thin before I did, I decided to find something else to fall back on. I decided to change my style. Working on my appearance would give me something to look at instead of the blasted scale.

At my fattest, I was always perfectly groomed. My hair was

perfect, the makeup was flawless. I had long nails and dark polish, and I wouldn't be caught dead in flat shoes. I felt thinner being taller.

If I went on a trip, the excess baggage I carried wasn't just around my waist. When you're fat, you need to take a lot of clothes with you. In the first place, your things wrinkle faster than thin people's. In the second, you never really feel comfortable in anything and you somehow think that changing into another outfit will make you feel thinner, which of course it won't. In the third place, you have to be prepared for every emergency. You can't get a pair of queen-sized taupe sandalfoot pantyhose in every corner of the globe. If you're in Alaska and someone finds an indoor, heated swimming pool, you want to have your skirted bathing suit with the built-in bra along, just in case no one can lend you one.

I wanted to create attention, so I went for the opposite of what people expected of me. Since I was a little thinner, I felt secure enough to pare down in every department. I went to the beauty shop and had my hair cut off and shaped into one of those styles you aren't supposed to bother with. Off came the nail polish and half the nail tips. The silk dresses went to the Salvation Army. I adopted a disguise: tennis shoes and slacks, shirts with the tails tucked in. No one would believe it was me.

Then I started to change my look every time I started getting sick of myself, mostly with makeup and hairstyles. I bought a couple of inexpensive wigs to make the change more dramatic. One week I was carefree, the next careerwoman, and then I went back to glamorous. I kept up the routine for months. My friends started calling me Sybil, but the trick kept me going.

About a month after I had started the diet, I felt secure enough to get rid of all my fat clothes. A lot of them had the original price tags on them. (But not the size tags: I always removed those immediately.) In the group were smaller-sized clothes that I had intended to wear after I lost weight. They were now too large.

There came a point when not a single thing in my closet fit. Everything was too big. I treated myself to some new clothes. I know it's a bit of a waste, but I don't think you should keep running around in size 20's when you're down to 16's. Buy yourself a couple pairs of inexpensive pants and shirts that fit to wear in the interim, and remind yourself of the money you've saved by cutting down on the eating.

I was continuing to cook for my family during the diet. In the past, I had had a lot of trouble keeping myself from sticking my finger into the cookpot and sampling. Now that had become less of a problem. I was making a conscious effort not to do that, and I wasn't cooking the kinds of dishes that lend themselves to that kind of sampling. You don't stick your finger into a broiled fillet of bluefish. Even after I went off the rigidly structured part of the program. I liked to plan my meals in advance, particularly the dinners. I got out a pad and paper and my calorie counter and I figured out what I was going to eat for the week. It made my shopping easier, of course.

In the beginning, I repeated a lot of the foods I'd eaten during the first two weeks, mostly because the nutritionist Dr. Joel was working with had made up some delicious menus. As I started feeling more comfortable about making intelligent choices, I branched out.

My family actually liked the new system. We had been eating a lot of the same foods over and over again, with a lot of beef as the main course. My tendency was to switch over to chicken, since that was a good low-calorie food, but the nutritionist suggested I vary the menu for my sake and the family's. So I found some new options. One night it would be shrimp, the next night something else. Sherm and Andrew told me they'd be looking forward to what we were having next.

Fortunately, I didn't have the problem my friends told me about. Their husbands just didn't want to eat the kinds of foods their wives prepared when they were on diets. Of course, my first reaction is that if the guy won't give up his mashed potatoes and deep-fried chicken for you, leave him. Doesn't he know that both of you will benefit when you're looking better? Also, if you're healthier you're probably going to be around a lot longer, and if he really cares about you, he should be all for that, too.

But I can't say I didn't have my problems with being sabotaged. It happens in marriages where the wife or husband has a weight problem and the thin partner says, "Let's go eat." He knows it makes you happy. I don't think the partner is doing it to be mean or malicious. There's a lot of love involved. "Hey, you've done a good job now, and you've lost some weight, so eat the ice cream."

The same thing happened when we went to my mother's house. Sundays at my mother's have always been an event for me, my sister, and two brothers. We just let it all hang out, and we did a good job of eating. This particular Sunday I remember was Mother's Day, and there were several kinds of cake on the table and I was going to have a little portion. It really did satisfy me to have just a couple of forkfuls. Suddenly I heard, "Oh, Mary Ellen, you should have a nice piece. It's Mother's Day."

The reaction is to get mad, until you realize you're being coaxed by somebody who believes the cake will make you feel good. Sure it will. For as long as it's in your mouth. But now you have to start dealing with the long term.

That Sunday, I posed for a lot of pictures, which I had been doing all along. Pictures serve two very important purposes: They help show you that you are getting thinner, and that you aren't thin yet. Those Mother's Day photos were a kind of landmark occasion for me, becuase I posed next to a lot of normal-sized people. And yet when I looked at the photos, for the first time the people in them didn't seem to have limbs like Olive Oyl compared to mine.

I had seen a woman on television who lost 150 pounds on a natural food diet. The show pictured her at her top weight and then at her goal weight. At the end, she didn't look as good as you would think, because her body was not toned; she hadn't done any exercise. She looked like a smaller version of a fat person, with the same roly-poly arms, just smaller dimensions. She wasn't taking up as much space, but she looked exactly the same. But I could see that wasn't happening to me. I felt very good.

I had to keep that image in my mind to keep going when I had a last major near-setback, about three-quarters of the way to goal. I met some friends in a restaurant who hadn't seen me for a very long time. I heard a lot of "Hey, Mary Ellen, I don't believe it," and "You look like a movie star." And then, halfway through lunch, someone said, "You know, you're really different. You're not fun anymore."

I thought, do I have to decide if I'm going to be fun or pretty? Because if it came down to it, I'd rather have a good time than look in the mirror. When I got down to goal, of course, I realized I could do both. At the same time.

Chapter 9

Fat No More

I am a firm believer that fat is the best method of birth control. Not until I lost weight did I start getting patted on the fanny again instead of on the back. I see myself in a completely different light now. I love to wear negligees, for instance. I used to hate them. Well, of course I did. It's hard to breathe deeply with passion when you're afraid the seams are about to go. Forget what you know about nylon being so strong they make parachutes out of it. There wasn't a nightgown built for the strain I put on it.

As I write this, I'm at my goal weight of 135 pounds. I've stabilized at it, and it seems to be the right weight for me. Now, I know there will be some anorexic type on the tube telling you and me that people five foot five should weigh 105, but I won't buy that. No, I'm not reed thin, but I'm in good shape. I think I look pretty good with my clothes on.

I go shopping for dresses and I don't need to ask a saleslady what makes me look good. I know when I'm looking good. Anytime the saleslady shows me a dress that looks as if you could fill it with foam pellets and make a beanbag chair out of it, I say, "Get that out of here." I want everything to be fitted. I absolutely will not wear another sack dress again, whether it's in fashion or not. I don't want to feel as if I have to cover myself up.

On the other hand, I'm not about to sign up for the Miss Nude America competition, either. I have my war wounds, my stretch marks. And sometimes that's hard for me to deal with. Let's face it, there probably isn't a person in America who wouldn't like to fiddle around with his or her proportions. Take a look at a lineup of dancers. These are people who are working out their bodies every day, who are in the best shape it's possible to be in. Yet some of them are a little too busty, or they have rib cages that are too big, or hips that are too wide, or their waists don't go in the way a waist should go. There are very few Bo Dereks or Farah Fawcetts out there.

Even if you suspect that you're contoured more like a soda bottle than an hourglass, there's no reason to work yourself up from the six-ounce bottle to the two-liter size. Even if you believe the setpoint theory, I think it's hard to accept the idea that 193 pounds is the setpoint that Nature intended for anyone under six feet tall.

When appearances are doled out, we each get a different color hair, eyes, skin—the whole bit. We even get a normal weight—normal, that is, for the individual. Even if yours doesn't put you in the fashion model category, so what? There aren't enough jobs to keep that many of us busy as fashion models. Maybe you got a little extra in the personality department, or you're a great mother.

Weight's only part of who you are. If you get yours down from a definitely obese 200 to 165 or from 165 to 145, be grateful and proud of what you've accomplished. Keep on the diet, stick with the walking. Your shape will definitely get better, whether or not you knock off more poundage. It's not how many pounds you weigh, anyway—it's whether those pounds are fat or lean muscle that determines how you look.

The important thing about getting on the Help Yourself program is that it's for life. You may see me somewhere eating a burger and fries, but you won't see me let a week go by without exercising for at least five days. I have had weekends when I've eaten to excess—not pigging out like in the old days, but eating more than I needed. When I was going on and off my fad diets, if I ate a little extra, my weight would shoot up five or six pounds. Now, it goes up just a little, and as soon as I notice that weight gain, I do something about it. I still find it difficult not to try and fast it off, but I have made a commitment to my body never to do that again. I do as Dr. Joel suggests: I cut back 400 calories, and keep walking, and that always corrects the situation within a couple of days.

I also keep a daily record of what I've eaten even when I'm overdoing it. It doesn't seem like a nuisance anymore. It's part of my daily routine, like brushing my teeth, and thanks to all the practice I had looking up calories, I'm now pretty familiar with the information. I can gauge the count of almost everything I eat and keep myself in check. Of course, now that my metabolism is working like a normal person's, I can pretty much eat what I like, and that's a real pleasure.

I was amazed to discover that I had actually worn out two pairs of walking shoes. I've worn out high heels before—with all that weight on them, I'm surprised I didn't grind them right down into stumps—but I can't get over the walking shoes. I'm thinking of having them bronzed to use as planters or doorstops. They'll be souvenirs.

My other souvenirs are in the photo album. I look at those photographs, and I have a hard time realizing that person was me. I think of myself as a thin person now; I've stopped making those fat jokes that I was the butt of.

I can't help thinking, How did I let myself go? when I look at those pictures, but I try not to blame myself. I tried to control my weight, but like most of the public, I was a victim of deception and hype dished out by a lot of so-called diet experts.

I got sick of hearing about weight loss and talking about it. Find another hobby, I said to myself. But no matter where I went, someone would be talking about losing weight, and then somebody else would beam down with some other "miracle diet" she heard about or read about or some gypsy in the street thrust in her hands.

They have a lot of different names, but I call them the Fool Yourself diets. They have about as much basis in reality as any other science fiction. Remember the movie *Invasion of the Body Snatchers*? Well, I was waiting for the invasion of the fat snatchers. Sorry, folks. They're not coming.

So I felt it was time somebody wrote a book that told the truth. No magic formula. No gimmicks. Just the assurance that it works. It takes a lot of effort, but I learned to Help Myself. And you can learn to Help Yourself, too.

Part Two

Help Yourself: The Program

Chapter 10

If You Really Want to Help Yourself, Read This Part

I'm now going to explain why the Help Yourself program works and why you should follow it (though, of course, you should check with your doctor before you start).

If you're like me, you want to rush past this section and get right to the diet. You don't want to be educated. You want to be thinner. Forget it. The diet is the least important part of this program. The diet alone is not what's going to make you lean and fit. That will happen only if you stay on the full program, and the only way you'll be really convinced that it's important to stay on it is to read what comes next. Then you'll know why the Help Yourself program will get that fat off and keep it off—and why any scheme that doesn't combine a well-balanced food plan with an exercise program (with a little bit of habit changing) will not.

It doesn't matter who comes onto the scene next—some guy telling you to dine on tree bark because it's high in fiber or a woman plugging the Miss Universe I Love the Galaxy diet or yet another doctor swearing on his stethoscope that you can lose weight following his magic plan that involves combining foods that rhyme—save your money. If you go on another one of those crazy diets, you're going to fail. Oh, you may lose a few pounds, but, ultimately, you'll gain them back. Ninety-eight percent of dieters do. Then you'll feel guilty, get depressed, and start eating—and keep right on until the next crackpot scheme comes out.

Let me tell you the truth, which most of the diet book authors in the past have not. If any diet you go on isn't based on the principles I'm about to explain, it can't work.

Here's Why You're Likely to Be Fat

- It may be genetic
- It may be physiological

First the Good News

It's not your fault you're fat. Some people think fat people are just self-indulgent slobs who have no willpower. Most of the fat people I know display an amazing amount of willpower each time they start a new diet; they may eventually fail, but they make some awfully good tries. Other people think it's a mental problem: Fat people are mental wrecks who head for the refrigerator every time they have a mood swing.

In 1980, the American Psychological Association got you off the hook. They issued an announcement that obesity is a physical disorder; it is not linked to a psychological problem. You may sometimes eat for emotional reasons—even thin people do—but that's okay. It's a problem, but you don't need years of therapy to uncover some dark spot in your psyche that's pointing you to the Oreos. Congratulations, sort of. You're not nuts; you're just fat. Why did you overeat so much that you got fat?

Your Genes Made You Do It

You're not used to thinking of your weight as a trait like your hair or your skin, but it is. Forty percent of children who have one overweight parent will have a weight problem themselves. Eighty percent of children with two overweight parents will. One reason for this may be that you pick up your parents' habit of overeating. But there also seems to be a genetic influence on your weight.

Being fat is always connected with how much you exercise. Researchers at Harvard noticed that even in infancy, there is a difference in how much individuals move. Babies who moved the most were the least likely to be overweight, even though they also ate the most. Babies who ate the least and moved the least were fattest. (I thought it was also interesting that babies of rat mothers who exercised while pregnant had a lot more muscle fibers in their bodies than other rat babies. If your mother didn't exercise, here's something else you can blame on her.)

Also, how fat you are is determined both by how many fat cells you have and how large they are. How many you have seems to be determined by heredity. You acquire most of the fat cell supply during your first two years, with an additional supply coming in at adolescence. (Pimples and fat: No wonder the teen years are so miserable.) Some unfortunate people have both a lot of fat cells and large fat cells. While you can shrink fat cells, as I did, you can never reduce the number, and having a lot means you tend to be a fat person.

In addition, some people's bodies have more of a special ingredient that helps them burn their food faster than you and I. It's called brown fat, and if you haven't heard of brown fat it's because scientists have only confirmed that it exists in adults within the last three years. (It exists in newborns to help maintain body temperature.) It's not something you'd notice anyway, since the largest deposit in your body is between your shoulder blades and it takes a thermogram to find it. Nobody yet knows what determines how much brown fat you have. Perhaps it's genetic. One theory postulates that it can be increased during a particular period of overfeeding during infancy. Back off from those baby food jars anyway: If you start overfeeding junior at the wrong period during infancy, he'll get an excess of the plain old white fat we all know and loathe.

Studies of people who matched in every respect (such as body size, amount of activity, and food intake) have shown that one might lose as much as twice as much body heat as the other during metabolism, and by losing that heat they burn off extra calories. In other words, people with a lot of brown fat can eat twice as much as other people—and not gain weight. Conversely, a lack of brown fat might make you gain weight easily—but that's not been proven yet.

Finally, there may be something wrong with your body's regulatory system that explains why you and the guy next to you have eaten the same amount but he's ready to quit and you aren't. Your stomach and blood sugar may be sending the message "Enough already," but for reasons scientists can't yet explain, it isn't getting through to your brain. A Cornell University Medical College study turned up a substance produced in the small intestine that may signal when you've had enough to eat. Obese rats have less of this substance than nonobese rats, and the same may be true in humans.

Even a specific craving for carbohydrates, which seems to affect women more than men, may have a chemical explanation. In most people, a brain chemical called serotonin increases after a small amount of carbohydrates are eaten, and the person stops craving more. In some fat people, serotonin activity stays too low.

Your Body May Have a Naturally High Weight

Some experts believe that your body has a natural weight or setpoint, which they describe as the weight your body reaches when you aren't counting calories. You may want to weigh 130, but your body's trying to get to 160. William Bennett, M.D., and Joel Gurin, who outlined this theory in *The Dieter's Dilemma*, explain that dieting is like pulling against a spring: You struggle to lose weight while your body struggles to keep it on. Perhaps this problem is linked to a substance called lipoprotein lipase (LPL). Obese people have more LPL in their blood. LPL levels go down during dieting, but return to high levels during maintenance.

Remedies

What does this mean to you? Until there's a pill that can reverse the effect of whatever it is in your body that made you move too little, produce too many fat cells or too little brown fat, or causes chemical imbalances, you've got a problem. Just like you've got a problem with hair that's mousy brown or skin that's too dry. But you change your hair color if you don't like it, and you do something about your skin. And if you're fat, there's no reason to stay at home crying into your bag of cookies. Even the setpoint theorists say you can change your setpoint. You *can* do something about your weight problem. It must be done over a period of time, and it will be harder for you than the rest of the (thin) world. But *it can be done.* I'm living proof.

Why Fad Diets Do You In

* No fad diet is based on the critical "energy equation."
* Fad diets make your system sluggish and promote eventual weight *gain.*
* Fad diets increase the amount of fat in your body—even if you lose weight.
* The more fat there is on your body, the harder it is to get fit and lean.
* Your "weight problem" is actually a "fat problem" and you can even be a *thin* fat person.

Input and Outgo

The energy you derive from the food you put into your body (input) and the energy you spend in keeping your body alive and moving (outgo) are the two parts of the "energy equation" that determine your weight.

Fad diets concentrate your attention on input—what you do or don't eat. You eat grapefruit, or eggs, or cottage cheese, or you may even count calories, and presto! The weight will come off. This approach makes the assumption that everyone's body works the same, which, of course, is not true.

Think of a car. How much fuel it requires doesn't depend on the size or style of the car but on the efficiency of the engine. Human beings are living things, so every part of them needs food for energy—that's why a 220-pound linebacker needs more food than a 110-pound secretary. But even among people of the same size, there is a variation in how much a body stores and how much it burns up.

Common sense tells you that to lose weight, you must take in less food than you need. Even "eat all you want" diets, which always restrict you to a set list of foods, are based on reduced caloric intake; it's been found that no matter what you're eating on a restricted plan, you soon get bored and eat less than usual.

Fad diets concentrate on reduced input, but never concern themselves with the other half of the energy equation: how you burn off that energy. The way to do it is through exercise. I know you've heard about how long you have to walk to burn off the calories in one apple, but, as I will explain, exercise does a great deal more than use up a certain number of calories.

Fad Dieting Made Your Problem Worse

If you have a genetic tendency to be fat, you probably went on your first diet around the time you started noticing the opposite sex. That's when you first got into trouble. Here's how:

You lost lean muscle. Let's say you lost twenty pounds. About half of it was water. Sorry, folks, but that's the truth. About five pounds was fat. And five pounds was healthy, lean muscle. More about the consequences of that later.

You slowed down your metabolic rate. Your metabolic rate is the rate at which you use energy (food you have eaten or food you stored as fat) and generate heat (a by-product of the process of using energy). When you're tested to find your *basal* metabolic rate, that's the rate at which you're burning food while at rest.

Dr. Joel explained to me that when there's a drop in food intake, the body, which resists weight loss because it wants to keep itself intact, starts to burn the food more slowly. The effect lasts for several weeks, possibly longer. No one knows for sure.

End-of-the-diet weight gain. By taking in less than your body needs to maintain itself, you cause your body to become fatigued. At the end of this diet, two things happen:

One: The fatigue and depression of dieting almost automatically cause you to crave more food and then to overeat.

Two: Your metabolism is still working at a lower rate, yet you're eating as much or possibly more than when you began the diet. Experimenters starved laboratory rats for a while, then put them back on their normal diet. During the first week of eating normally, they gained more than twenty times the weight of animals who had been fed the same amount without being starved first. (There is an additional theory that this may also be linked to levels of LPL, the substance I mentioned a few pages back.) When I found out about this, it was the first time I'd ever felt badly for a rat.

This is why any fat loss program should get your metabolism working properly by gradually increasing the amount of food you take in as you lose weight. Instead of being trained to work more slowly as you eat less (that's what happened on a fad diet), on the Help Yourself program, your metabolism is slowly adjusted to working harder and harder. When you've reached goal, it's "set" to burn off the calories you're taking in.

Fat Makes You Fatter

I have mentioned that on a fad diet you lose lean muscle. If you don't exercise, you replace that lean muscle with fat. Here's what that means to your body:

Fat tissue is, for the most part, inactive. It carries on some metabolic processes, but at a low rate. It uses few calories. Lean tissue, on the other hand, is active muscle, and it does use calories. The more of your body that is made up of muscle, the more calories you use up in doing everything from breathing to walking. And vice-versa.

If you regained your weight after the fad diet, you probably continued to eat the same amount as before you dieted. Even if the scale stayed the same, since you didn't exercise, your body contained a higher percentage of fat than before, so it actually needed less food. The result was you got fatter.

When you're fat, your body doesn't burn fats properly. Everything you eat, you will remember from your health classes, is made up of protein, carbohydrates, or fats. When you need energy, your body gets it by burning carbohydrates first and turning them into glucose. Since only a relatively small amount of glucose is kept on hand in your body (after a very short time it is put into storage in the liver) the body quickly uses it up and then dips into its fat stores.

Humans and animals store any excess food as fats. Camels, who store fat in their humps, convert the fat to water during their long desert trips, which inspired me to a poem:

> The camel stores his fat in humps.
> Yours is in unsightly bumps.
> The camel's fat helps quench his thirst.
> Yours just makes you look your worst.

The unfair fact is that people who are fat do not give up their stores of fat easily, the way lean and fit people do. If you're in good shape, you can dip into your fat stores readily. If you're not, you cannot. You need energy, though, so you get hungry. That's why fat people often want to eat after exercise and thin people do not.

Eventually, the fat stores of unfit people will break down, but only over a long period of time. Fat bodies were designed to exist during times of famine; but in a civilization of abundance, like the United States, they just get fatter.

Being fat predisposes you to getting fatter. The metabolic processes of obese people are altered. Their fat cells store more fat more easily than those of thin people. The problem you have just gets—pardon the expression—larger.

The Scales Don't Tell the Whole Story

Like most people, I tactfully refer to my "weight" problem. Enough of this beating around the bush. The problem is fat. There are even *thin* fat people running around. Dressed, they look like skinny people. Undressed, you'll be relieved to know, they look like you and I. You've seen them. They weigh what the charts say they should, but they have narrow shoulders, no waist, and thick thighs—any or all of the above. They keep their weight down by eating very little.

Many women claim that they eat hardly anything and they're still not lean and fit, and that's true. Most American women eat less than 1600 calories a day, which is about right if you weigh 120 pounds—ideally, you sustain your weight by eating about 14 calories per pound—yet most American women weigh more than 120. They're not in shape, and they've wrecked their body's system through fad dieting. Ideally, a woman's body should be composed of about 22 percent fat (men's should be 17 percent) and yet many are higher—up to 45 percent. The only real way to know what percent fat you're made of is by having some rather sophisticated testing done, but you can get an idea by doing a little pinch test.

This might be easier if you ask a friend to do it. I hope you can find a close and supportive friend. There are four spots to test:

a. Take a vertical pinch from the back of your arm midway between your shoulder and elbow.
b. Take a horizontal pinch about an inch below your waist and an inch to the right of your belly button.
c. Take a diagonal pinch just above your hipbone.
d. Take a vertical pinch from the front of your upper thigh.

If you have any doubts about whether you're fat, pinch a skinny friend and compare yourself to her. Or take my word for it: If you've got an inch in at least two of those places, you're too fat. Or, if you absolutely want to know the worst, you can send away for a little gadget that measures these skinfolds (that's what they're called in the medical biz) by mailing $6.95 to Fitness Finders, Box 507, Spring Arbor, MI 49283. You'll get a less expensive version of the instrument doctors use.

When I heard that men's metabolic rates were higher than women's, I didn't think it was fair. I even considered having a sex-change operation. Then someone pointed out that men burn their food faster because they have less fat on their bodies.

Increasing the percent of body muscle, and decreasing the percent of fat as a result, is vital in a program that will make you lean and fit. The only way that can be done is through exercise. That's why Dr. Joel made exercise such an important and necessary part of the Help Yourself plan.

Why the Help Yourself Plan Is the Only Type That Can Work

• What a successful plan must combine
• Why not eating a well-balanced diet is dangerous

63

- Why eating several times a day helps you lose weight
- Why exercise is critical to a fat loss program
- Why it's necessary to change your habits

How a Fat Loss Program Must Work

A plan that works must include a diet that modifies your intake; exercise, to change the regulators of the outgo; and a set of guidelines to help you change your eating habits.

The Eating Plan Must Start with a Well-Balanced Diet

A government committee studying nutrition reported that a person should take in a daily mixture of 15–20 percent protein, 50–65 percent carbohydrates, and 20–30 percent fats. You should avoid excessive sugar and fats. You should also eat four times a day and not skip a meal—not even breakfast. We know how many times you have heard all this. But have you ever had an explanation?

Eating the proper balance keeps you from getting hungry and also keeps you healthy. As you now know, your body first uses the carbohydrates you have eaten, and then, when it goes through the limited store of these, it goes to the fats for fuel. Fats are broken down last, and they help give you that full feeling that prevents you from overeating. So they should be included on any diet in modest amounts.

If you aren't taking in enough carbohydrates when you eat, you interfere with the normal sequence. If you run out of carbohydrates quickly, your body will start breaking down protein before it goes to fat. The protein being used comes from muscle, which is meant to be part of your body's structure, not a source of energy. If your body is desperate, it will break down even organs, like the heart muscle. When you lost weight rapidly, as you do in most fad diets, that is always an indication that muscle is being lost instead of fat. (Fat contains many more calories per pound than muscle; it takes longer to lose a pound of fat than muscle. Also, muscle, unlike fat, is associated with a lot of water, which leaves your body along with the muscle.) Experimenters put some animals on fad diets and others on sound diets and discovered that animals on fad diets lost weight sooner, but those on well-balanced diets eventually lost as much weight and more body fat (instead of muscle tissue). After a fad diet, you may weigh less—but you have a higher percentage of body fat.

A too-rich diet raises your setpoint. Bet you're not surprised.

When laboratory animals are fed food that's fatty and sugary, they eat more of it. Rats, which don't usually become fat, *will* gain weight on what's called a cafeteria diet—that's peanut butter, sandwich cookies, fruit punches, and all the other things that taste good and are bad for you. Foods in that category are low in nutritional value, so Nature made sure that animals would get all the nutrition necessary from "junk food" by overeating it on the rare occasions when they'd come across it. When Nature set this up, of course, she didn't know bags full of candy corn and gallons of ice cream loaded with butterfat would one day be as close as the nearest supermarket.

Eating frequently helps you stay fit. There is some evidence that when you eat only one big meal a day, you store more food than if you eat several times a day; scientists don't know why this is true, but your fat-storing pathways seem to operate better when you eat once daily. Also, the very act of eating seems to burn off calories, which is why sometimes eating regularly is more effective than fasting. The name for this phenomenon is *diet-induced thermogenesis.*

What Is Thermogenesis?

Your body uses food in three ways. Some of it is used to keep your system going—to do everything from breathing to moving. Some food goes into storage. And some of it is lost as heat. That process is called thermogenesis. (Think of the heat generated by almost every working machine you can think of.) One example of thermogenesis is heat given off from eating. Think of the advice to starve a fever—the act of eating raises the amount of heat produced by your body, which is not desirable when your temperature is already elevated. Shivering is another kind of thermogenesis; it happens when your body tries to make you warmer.

If you're too fat, you want to increase thermogenesis so that your body loses more food as heat and stores less food as fat. There are two influences on body thermogenesis. One is the brown fat I mentioned earlier, but no one knows how to increase the amount of brown fat yet. The other influence is skeletal muscle (as opposed to organ muscle, like the heart). We do know how to do something about skeletal muscle—you can build it up, and thus build up the thermogenetic effect, through exercise.

Exercise Is as Important as Diet

Exercise has several important roles. One, it increases the amount of skeletal muscle. A person whose body has a higher percentage of lean muscle loses more calories thermogenetically, as heat. Besides, increasing your skeletal muscle as you diet will prevent that gaunt look that makes everyone tell you you look "too thin" while they tell Bo Derek she's just right. Dieters who look gaunt have simply lost too much muscle. (Besides, when you don't use your muscle, part of that muscle fiber just won't grow back. If muscles are out of shape, they lose the "girdle" effect on your layers of fat tissue.)

The idea is to replace fat with muscle. My mother warned me if I exercised, my fat would turn into muscle. Well, now I have something to tell you, Mother. Fat has about as much chance of turning into muscle as Kermit does of turning into a prince. Your muscle looks like a nicely marbled steak: Your goal is to burn up the fat and retain the muscle. In fact, all you can do is burn the fat: You can't change it into muscle.

Interestingly, since muscle weighs more than fat, as you build up muscle, you may weigh a bit more on the scale, but your clothes will be getting looser. (Reducing your calories while you exercise will, of course, result in a net weight loss.)

The other role of exercise is to increase your metabolic rate. You used to be told that such and such exercise used up so many calories. Actually, it has a much more important effect. Now scientists have discovered that exercise can speed up your metabolic rate for as long as twenty-four hours. Long after the exercise is over, your body is burning up calories more quickly while you're moving normally and even as you sleep.

As a bonus, scientists also think that exercise within an hour or so after a meal speeds up diet-induced thermogenesis.

The right kind of exercise is steady and calls for a lot of endurance. Since you're not trying to build up muscle, but rather to burn off fat, you need what's called an "aerobic exercise." Of them all, for reasons soon explained, we've chosen walking.

Finally, you need to change some of your habits. Your regulatory system may be off. Researchers speculate that is why fat people so often depend on outside clues (seeing that the clock reads noon) rather than inner ones (feeling their stomachs growling) to move them to eat.

In order to lose weight, you must replace some of these clues with new ones. If passing the bakery is enough to trigger you to buy an éclair, then you must avoid passing the bakery. You must consciously substitute new, helpful habits for old, harmful ones. Dr. Joel indicated some ways to change my behavior, and I discovered some of my own. You can read them in the pages that follow.

Now That You Understand the Reasons Behind the Help Yourself Plan, Here Is a Brief Description

THE EIGHT-STEP HELP YOURSELF DIET PLAN

Step #	How Long	Daily Diet	Exercise
1	ONE WEEK	1000 calories (Menus provided)	20 minutes moderate walking, 5 times weekly
2	ONE WEEK or until within four pounds of goal	1000 calories (Menus provided)	30 minutes moderate walking, 5 times weekly
3	UNTIL WITHIN FOUR POUNDS OF GOAL	1000 calories (Self-selection)	60 minutes including warmup, cool down, 30 minutes of brisk walking 5 times weekly
4	UNTIL WITHIN TWO POUNDS OF GOAL	1200 calories (Self-selection)	Continue Step #3
5	UNTIL AT GOAL	1400 calories (Self-selection)	Continue Step #3
6	UNTIL ONE POUND *BELOW* GOAL	1600 calories (Self-selection)	Continue Step #3

| 7 | UNTIL TWO POUNDS *BELOW* GOAL | 1800 calories (Self-selection) | Continue Step #3 |
| 8* | UNTIL YOU HAVE GAINED 1-2 POUNDS | 2000 calories or more (Self-selection) | Continue Step #3 |

---

*In Step #8, add calories in 200-calorie increments weekly until you have gained 1-2 pounds. Determine your caloric needs by picking a midpoint between the caloric intake on which you were losing and the caloric intake on which you are now gaining. You may find you are comfortable at a goal weight higher than originally anticipated since your body is in better shape. *You are now stabilized at your goal weight.* You must continue to exercise.

If, for any reason, you gain, drop your calorie intake 400 calories daily until you are back to goal weight. Never return to the 800- or 1000-calorie level.

Note:

- A diet diary *must* be kept throughout. See Part Three: Second Helpings (p. 206) for sample.
- Drink six to eight glasses of water or enough to pass at least a quart of urine daily.
- Ask your doctor to recommend a multivitamin to take daily. Take it along with the meal in which you have the most fat, since certain vitamins are only absorbed in the presence of fat.
- If you feel tired or feel not yourself, check with your doctor.

Goal weight may be determined from the latest Metropolitan Life Insurance Company height and weight chart, published December 1982, which you may get by writing to Metropolitan Life, Attention: Statistical Bureau, 1 Madison Plaza, New York, N.Y. 10010. Note that weights listed are higher than in the past. Also, since you will be more muscular than you used to be (and muscle, as you know, weighs more than fat), you might find yourself revising your personal goal weight upward as you stay on the program. You may look and feel better at a higher weight than you had originally planned.

A Two-Week Shopping List for the 1000-Calorie Diet

To make it easy for you to start your diet, I've made up a shopping list. It includes everything you'll need over the first two weeks on your diet. In order to vary the menu, I've included some items you can't buy in very small quantities, so you may have extra of some items. Freeze it or *give it away* if you must.

Meat and Fish	Week #1	Week #2
Tuna, canned, water-pack	1 can (6½ oz.)	1 can (6½ oz.)
Shrimp, canned		1 can (7 oz.)
Chicken, skinned and boned breast	11 oz.	8 oz.
Sirloin, lean	5 oz.	6½ oz.
Hamburger, lean		4 oz.
Pork steak, boned and trimmed fillet	5 oz.	5 oz.
Red snapper	7 oz.	
OR		
Scallops	6 oz.	
Flounder or sole, fillet	6 oz.	12 oz.
Cornish hen	16 oz.	
Shrimp, fresh, in shell	8 oz.	
Canadian bacon	2 oz.	1 oz.
Lamb chops, loin or rib		2 5-oz. chops

Dairy Products		
Skim milk	2 pints	1 pint
Eggs	3	4
Vanilla or lemon low-fat yogurt	8 oz.	8 oz.
Plain low-fat yogurt	8 oz.	12 oz.
Parmesan cheese	small can	
Butter or margarine	¼ lb.	

Starches	Week #1	Week #2
Unsweetened whole grain cereal (choose from calorie counter, p. 97)	1 box	
Oatmeal	1 box	
Thin-sliced whole wheat bread	7 slices	12 slices
Whole wheat melba toast	1 box	
Rice, white converted	1 box	
Egg noodles	1 box	
Popcorn	1 can, unpopped	
Waffles, frozen jumbo (Downyflake or Aunt Jemima)	2 waffles	2 waffles

Fruit and Vegetables—Fresh

	Week #1	Week #2
Medium bananas (6″)	3	1
Strawberries	2 cups (approx. 12 oz.)	1½ cup (approx. 9 oz.)
Medium peaches (if not in season, substitute tangerine, ½ pear, or ½ C. chunk unsweetened pineapple in its own juice)	3	4
Cantaloupe (if not in season, substitute ½ grapefruit for each ¼ melon)	1	1
Medium apples (2¼″ diameter)	5	6
Medium oranges	3	2
Grapefruit		1
Green pepper	1	1
Tomatoes, medium	3	3
Green beans	3 oz.	5½ oz.
Beets (2″ diameter, 3.5 oz. apiece)	2	
Zucchini (1 medium, about 6 oz.)		1
Celery	2 stalks	2 stalks
Broccoli	4 med. spears	8 med. spears
Acorn squash, 1 small (1 lb.)	½	½
Carrots, medium (1″ × 5½″)	5	3
Cucumber	1	

Fruit and Vegetables *(cont'd.)*	**Week #1**	**Week #2**
Asparagus (frozen if necessary)	10 spears	
Mushrooms	6 oz.	6 oz.
Lettuce, small head	1	1
Baking potato (2½″ diameter, approx. 5½ oz.)	2	1
Sweet potato (4 oz.)		2
Parsley (optional)	1 small bunch	
Chives (optional)	1 bunch	
Garlic	1 clove	

Other

	Week #1	
Raisins	small package	
Unsweetened applesauce	1 8-oz. jar	
Frozen orange juice concentrate	1 small can	
Lemon juice	1 squeeze bottle	
Prepared mustard (optional)	1 small jar	
Vegetable oil	1 bottle	
Low-calorie salad dressing (1 T. = 20 calories)	1 bottle	
Diet mayonnaise	1 jar	
Dry mustard		
Paprika		
Ginger		
Cinnamon		
Nutmeg		

Fourteen Days of 1000-Calorie* Menus

DAY 1

Breakfast

¾ C. unsweetened whole grain creal	70
½ C. skim milk	45
½ medium banana	45
	160

Lunch

Sandwich made with:

2 slices thin whole wheat bread	80
½ 6½-oz. can water-packed tuna	110
½ T. diet mayonnaise	20
½ tomato	15
lettuce leaf	0
¼ cantaloupe	35
½ C. skim milk	45
	305

Dinner

5 oz. (raw weight) lean sirloin, broiled	300
1 potato, baked	90
with 1 tsp. margarine or butter	35
2 oz. mushroom, cooked	15
5 fresh asparagus spears, steamed	20
2 medium carrots, steamed	40
	500

Snack

1 medium apple	80
	1040

---

*A brief calorie counter is found in Part Three: Second Helpings, p. 202. Calories have been rounded off to the nearest whole number. You'll see that calories don't come out to exactly 1000 every day—the total on some days will be slightly under and on others slightly over.

Helpful Hints for Day #1

- Slice the remaining half of banana from this morning's breakfast, wrap tightly in an airtight bag, then freeze. Tomorrow evening mix it with the vanilla yogurt and strawberries for a nice ice-cream type dessert.
- If you must use a leftover can of tuna in oil, be sure you rinse it under cold running water and pat dry with paper towels before eating.
- Cooked meat shrinks. I've given you specific raw weights to buy throughout the fourteen days, but you might want to know the rules of thumb for future use. Beef: Expect 1 ounce shrinkage for every 4 ounces purchased. Chicken: A 6-ounce piece with bones will yield 3 ounces of cooked meat. Fish: 10 ounces will give you 5 ounces of fillet.
- For mushrooms in a light gravy: Wash just before you use them by rinsing briefly in cool water, then blot with a damp paper towel. Put in a frying pan with enough water to cover them half-way, add paprika and pepper, and simmer briefly until mushrooms are soft.

Comments from Mary Ellen on Day #1

- At first the portions may look very small to you. They did to me. I had never dealt with half-cup measurements in my life. I didn't know they existed. Let me assure you that once the food is on your plate, you'll be surprised. There'a a lot there.
- I felt full on 1000 calories because I was used to no breakfast, a light lunch, and then a six-hour dinner. When's the last time you ate three meals a day?
- If you experience true hunger, don't snack. Drink a couple of glasses of water or go for a walk. It'll soon disappear.
- And finally, congratulations on your good start at Helping Yourself. Keep going.

DAY 2

Breakfast
1 whole egg, poached	75
1 slice thin whole wheat bread	40
¼ cantaloupe	35
	150

Lunch
Mix together:
4 oz. plain yogurt	70
½ cucumber, diced	10
1 medium tomato	30
1 stalk celery, diced	10
½ green pepper, chopped	10
3 slices whole wheat melba toast	45
1 medium peach	40
	215

Dinner
6 oz. skinned and boned breast of chicken, baked	300
1 C. fresh broccoli (4 medium spears)	40
with 1 tsp. margarine or butter and	35
1 tsp. Parmesan cheese	10
½ C. cooked rice	80
with 1 tsp. margarine or butter and	35
½ tsp. chopped parsley	0
	500

Snack
½ medium banana, sliced	45
½ C. sliced strawberries	25
mixed with 2 oz. vanilla yogurt	50
	120
	985

Helpful Hints for Day #2

- When's the best time to buy eggs? Small and medium are most plentiful in the fall. Large eggs are cheaper and more available in the spring.
- The best-tasting cantaloupes should have no greenish cast to the skin. A ripe one will have a pleasant odor and will yield to slight finger pressure at the blossom end—the end opposite the stem.
- Have a cucumber to peel and can't find your potato peeler? Use a spatula-type cheese cutter to get the job done quickly.
- Cook tonight's chicken plus an additional 4 oz. to use for lunch tomorrow and Day #5.
- Don't buy chicken with brownish areas: It's been in the supermarket fridge too long or been stored improperly. Forget it, also, if the skin looks dry, purplish, bruised, or scaly.
- Keep parsley fresh and crisp by storing in a wide-mouth jar with a tight lid.
- Add artificial sweetener to the yogurt if you need a sweeter treat. Try different brands of yogurt, since they vary in consistency and tartness; but be sure to check the label for the calorie count.

*   *   *

DAY 3

Breakfast

¾ C. unsweetened whole grain cereal	70
½ C. skim milk	45
¼ cantaloupe	35
	150

Lunch

Salad made with:

diced cooked chicken (2 oz. raw)	100
1 medium apple, diced	80
1 stalk celery, diced	10
1 T. diet mayonnaise	40
¼ cucumber	5
served on lettuce leaves	0
2 slices whole wheat melba toast	30
	265

Dinner

6 oz. (raw weight) flounder or sole, baked or broiled with dash lemon	150
½ tomato, baked or broiled	15
with 1 T. Parmesan cheese	25
½ small acorn squash, baked	80
with 1 tsp margarine or butter	35
1½ oz. green beans	25
with 1 tsp. butter or margarine	35
½ C. strawberries, sliced, with	25
½ medium banana, sliced	45
	435

Snack

popcorn, 2 C., popped with ½ T. oil or 3 C. popped without oil	160
	950

Helpful Hints for Day #3

- Line the bottom of your lettuce crisper with paper towels to keep lettuce fresh and crisp longer. The paper towels absorb all the excess moisture.
- Strawberries can be kept firm for several days if you store them in a colander in the refrigerator, which allows the cold air to circulate around them. Don't hull them until they have been washed or they will absorb too much water and become mushy.
- Cooking a perfect fish is easy, if you remember this ten-minute rule—whether you're broiling, baking, simmering, poaching, or steaming fresh (not frozen) fish. A 1" thick piece takes ten minutes to cook. Add two minutes cooking time for every quarter inch above one inch, and subtract two minutes for every quarter inch below. Flounder, at about one-quarter inch, will cook in 3-4 minutes, 1¼" salmon in 12–13.
- Slice tomatoes vertically and the slices stay firm while baking.
- Lower-calorie popcorn: cover the pan bottom with salt instead of oil or butter. Heat the salt, then add the popcorn.

DAY 4

Breakfast

¾ C. unsweetened whole grain cereal	70
½ C. skim milk	45
½ C. strawberries	25
	140

Lunch

Sandwich made with:	
1 slice thin whole wheat bread	40
½ 6½-oz. can water-packed tuna	110
½ T. diet mayonnaise	20
1 T. Parmesan cheese (sprinkle on top and place sandwich under broiler or in microwave oven briefly)	25
1 medium apple	80
	275

Dinner

8 oz. shrimp (raw), peeled and deveined	200
(sauté in ½ T. vegetable oil with	50
1 clove minced garlic)	0
½ C. rice	80
Salad made with:	
½ small head lettuce	25
½ carrot, chopped	10
½ tomato, chopped	15
2 tsp. Parmesan cheese	15
1 T. low-calorie salad dressing	20
asparagus, fresh, 5 spears, steamed	20
	435

Snack

4 oz. plain yogurt with	70
1 sliced peach	40
	110
	960

Helpful Hints for Day #4

- Tuna in chunks or flakes is cheaper than solid but just as nutritious.

- After shelling and deveining shrimp, put them in a bowl and wash gently under cold, running water for half a minute. Next, rinse them in a colander under briskly running cold water for about three minutes. When cooked, they will almost crunch.
- Remove the tops of carrots before storing in the refrigerator. Tops drain the carrots of moisture, making them limp and dry.
- Asparagus, like lima beans, corn, and spinach, lose moisture fast. They should be refrigerated the moment you come home from the market.

* * *

DAY 5

Breakfast

1 slice thin whole wheat toast	40
1 whole egg, scrambled in nonstick pan	75
1 medium orange	80
	195

Lunch

Sandwich made with:

1 thin slice whole wheat bread	40
1 T. diet mayonnaise	40
Sliced chicken without skin (2 oz. raw weight)	100
Lettuce leaf	0
1 medium apple	80
	260

Dinner

7 oz. red snapper *or* 6 oz. scallops, broiled with lemon and paprika	190
½ C. egg noodles	100
2 beets, steamed	30
1 tsp. margarine or butter	35
1 sliced peach	40
	395

Snack

2 slices melba toast with	30
1 tsp. margarine or butter, sprinkled with cinnamon	35
4 oz. vanilla yogurt	100
	165
	1015

78

Helpful Hints for Day #5

- The larger apples have more than 80 calories; besides, small and medium fruits are generally tastier than large ones.
- Apples should be smooth, firm to the touch, and free of bruises. Avoid red apples that are greenish; pass by Golden Delicious apples that are very large and deeply yellow. Both are a sign of aging and mealiness.
- For silky-smooth scrambled eggs, start with a cool nonstick pan and cook eggs very slowly.
- Put aside beet greens in the freezer for eventual use. A whole cup is only 30 calories. Boil gently and chop like spinach.

* * *

DAY 6

Breakfast

¾ C. oatmeal	100
with 1 medium apple, chopped	80
and cinnamon to taste	0
½ C. skim milk	45
	225

Lunch

Salad made with:	
½ small head lettuce	25
½ green pepper, chopped	10
½ carrot, sliced	10
2 oz. mushroom, sliced	15
½ tomato, chopped	15
¼ cucumber, chopped	5
1 hard-boiled egg, chopped	75
1 T. low-calorie salad dressing	20
3 slices whole wheat melba toast	45
1 medium banana	90
	310

Dinner

5 oz. (raw weight) pork steak, broiled	300
1 medium potato, baked, with 1 tsp.	90
margarine or butter	35
1½ oz. green beans, steamed, with dash of	25
lemon	
	450

79

Snack

1 medium orange   80
                                                                            ————
                                                                            1065

Helpful Hints for Day #6

- Store apples alone. Apples tend to give off a gas that can make carrots bitter.
- You can substitute the Special Vinaigrette (see Formerly Fattening Meals in Part Three: Second Helpings) for low-calorie salad dressing.
- There's more to making hard-boiled eggs than you might think. Place eggs in a pan, cover with cold water, and pour in some vinegar or salt. The vinegar keeps the egg from oozing out if the shell cracks while cooking. Bring to a boil and remove from heat. Set in covered pan for twenty minutes. Drain off hot water. Now, shake the pan back and forth, causing the eggs to crack against the side. Cool with cold water and peel.
- Use an egg slicer to slice mushrooms uniformly and easily.
- Bumps on green string beans mean they are tough, so there is more waste. Select young, small ones.
- Rough, pitted skin may indicate that an orange is dry, so choose oranges with smooth, thin skin.

*   *   *

DAY 7

Brunch

2 medium waffles with	170
½ C. unsweetened applesauce	50
2 oz. Canadian bacon	90
¼ cantaloupe	40
	———
	350

Dinner

16 oz. Cornish hen (remove skin, eat all meat, 5 oz.)	250
(baste with 2 tsp. frozen orange juice	10
concentrate mixed with 1 tsp. water	0
and a dash of ginger if desired)	0

½ C. cooked rice with	80
½ tsp. margarine or butter	20
½ tsp. chopped parsley	0
2 oz. sliced mushrooms	15
2 carrots, steamed with	40
1 tsp. margarine or butter	35
1 medium orange, sliced	80
	530

Snack

2 oz. vanilla yogurt	50
½ medium banana, sliced	45
½ C. sliced strawberries	25
	120
	1000

Helpful Hints for Day #7

- Mix cinnamon, nutmeg, ginger, and cloves to taste if you want a spicier applesauce; or use pumpkin pie spice.
- To store unused orange juice concentrate, remove needed concentrate without thawing all the juice by running hot water over the outside of the can until concentrate is softened just enough to use. Then cover the top surface with plastic wrap and secure the top of can with a rubber band. Replace can in the freezer.
- Mushrooms won't get slimy if you refrigerate them in a brown paper bag. Paper allows the mushrooms to "breathe" while keeping in the humidity that keeps them fresh.
- Or, store mushrooms, already sliced, in your freezer.

DAY 8

Breakfast

1 slice thin whole wheat toast	40
1 tsp. margarine or butter	35
1 whole egg, scrambled with	75
1 T. skim milk	10
½ grapefruit	40
	200

Lunch

Sandwich made with:

1 thin slice whole wheat bread	40
3½ oz. canned shrimp (½ small can) drained	115
1 T. diet mayonnaise	40
lettuce leaf	0
1 medium peach	40
	235

Dinner

5 oz. (raw weight) sirloin, broiled	300
2 oz. mushrooms, cooked	15
½ C. egg noodles with	100
½ tsp. margarine or butter and	20
½ tsp. chopped parsley	0
2 carrots, steamed	40
	475

Snack

4 oz. plain yogurt with	70
2 tsp. frozen orange juice concentrate	10
½ medium banana, sliced	45
	125
	1035

Helpful Hints for Day #8

- To keep the other half grapefruit fresh, put it cut side down in a small bowl and refrigerate.
- Buy grapefruit that's heavy for its size (test in your palm) and thin-skinned. Pink looks pretty but tastes exactly like yellow and costs more.

- Store leftover canned shrimp in a tightly covered refrigerator dish or plastic bag, not in the can.
- Broil the remaining 1½ ounces of steak for lunch Day #9.
- When you buy carrots, buy them with tops off. They lose moisture through those pretty green leaves.

*   *   *

DAY 9

Breakfast

¾ C. oatmeal with	100
1 T. raisins, cinnamon, and nutmeg	30
½ C. skim milk	45
¼ cantaloupe	40
	215

Lunch

Sandwich made with:

1 slice thin whole wheat bread	40
1½ oz. (raw weight) sliced cooked sirloin	90
½ small tomato, sliced	15
1 tsp. mustard	5
lettuce leaf	0
1 medium apple	80
	230

Dinner

6 oz. sole or flounder, broiled or baked	150
½ small acorn squash, baked	80
topped with 1 tsp. margarine or butter	35
¼ tsp. cinnamon	0
Salad made with:	
½ small head lettuce	25
½ carrot, chopped	20
2 oz. mushrooms, sliced	15
1 T. low-calorie salad dressing	20
1 potato, baked	90
1 medium peach	40
	475

Snack

1 medium orange	80
	1000

Helpful Hints for Day #9

- Take the lumps out of cooked cereal by whipping with a wire whisk.
- Store raisins in a cool, dry place until you open the package, then put them in a plastic bag and store in the refrigerator.
- When selecting carrots, bear in mind that young, slender ones are usually sweeter. Thick carrots, deeper in color, are older and would be better for stews and soups.
- If tiny flies are buzzing around peaches (or cheeries or plums) don't buy them. It means the fruit is overripe. Don't buy when green, either. Peaches won't ripen at home.

*   *   *

DAY 10

Breakfast

2 slices whole wheat toast	80
4 oz. plain yogurt with	70
½ C. strawberries	25
1 tsp. orange juice concentrate	10
	185

Lunch

Salad made with:

½ small head lettuce	25
½ 6½-oz. can water-packed tuna	110
½ carrot, chopped	20
1 stalk celery, chopped	10
1 T. low-calorie salad dressing	20
1 medium apple	80
	265

Dinner

6 oz. (raw weight) boneless, skinless chicken breast, baked	300
1 zucchini (approx. 6 oz.), steamed,	20
topped with 1 tsp. Parmesan cheese	10
½ C. cooked rice with	80
1 tsp. margarine or butter	35
	445

84

Snack

2 oz. vanilla yogurt	50
1 peach, sliced	40
	90

985

Helpful Hints for Day #10

- An easy way to slice or chop carrots is to put the whole carrot inside the curve of a celery stalk. The carrot doesn't roll around—and you'll have both vegetables sliced or chopped at one time.
- Bake an additional 2 ounces (raw weight) of chicken to be used for lunch on Day #11.
- Realize that by cooking your own chicken, you are saving not only calories but also money. Prepared chicken costs four times as much as fresh.
- An easy way to peel peaches: Dip the fruit into boiling water for fifteen seconds, then dip into cold water (to prevent from cooking). The skin will slide right off.

*   *   *

DAY 11

Breakfast

¾ C. unsweetened whole grain cereal	70
½ C. skim milk	45
½ C. strawberries	25
	140

Lunch

Sandwich made with:

2 thin slices whole wheat bread	80
sliced chicken without skin (2 oz. raw weight)	100
½ tomato sliced	15
1 T. diet mayonnaise	40
lettuce leaf	0
1 medium apple	80
	315

DAY 11 (cont'd.)

Dinner

4 oz. lean hamburger, broiled	240
6 T. unsweetened applesauce	35
1 small sweet potato or yam, baked with	140
1 tsp. margarine or butter	35
2 oz. steamed green beans, with	30
1 tsp. margarine or butter	35
	515

Snack

1 medium orange	80
	1050

Helpful Hints for Day #11

• The tip of your potato peeler is great for removing the stems from strawberries. Just insert it underneath the stem cap, hold the cap with your thumb and lift off quickly and easily.
• Buy tomatoes with the stem attached. The tiny stem helps keep in moisture.
• Use a melon baller to core an apple half quickly and easily.
• You can cut the baking time by as much as half if you place potatoes on the oven rack and then place an iron pot over them.

* * *

DAY 12

Breakfast

1 waffle	85
1 tsp. margarine or butter	35
4 oz. vanilla yogurt	100
½ medium banana	45
	225

Lunch

Sandwich made with:

1 slice thin whole wheat bread	40
½ 6½-oz. can shrimp, drained	115
1 stalk celery, diced	10
1 T. diet mayonnaise	40
dash dry mustard	0
½ C. sliced strawberries	25
	230

Dinner

2 5-oz. (raw weight) broiled lamb chops	250
(eat *lean* meat only)	
½ C. rice, steamed, with	80
1 tsp. margarine or butter	35
1 small tomato, sliced, with	30
1 T. low-calorie salad dressing	20
4 spears broccoli	20
	435

Snack

4 oz. plain yogurt with	70
2 tsp. frozen orange juice concentrate	10
1 medium peach, sliced	40
	120
	1005

Helpful Hints for Day #12

- Canned shrimp lose their "canned" taste if you soak them for fifteen minutes in two tablespoons of vinegar and a teaspoon of sherry.
- They may look pretty, but skip the giant strawberries. Sweetest are medium-sized, no larger than a quarter.
- Green tomatoes ripen in a cool, dark corner.

*   *   *

DAY 13

Breakfast

1 slice thin whole wheat bread	40
with 1 tsp. margarine or butter	35
1 egg, poached	75
1 medium apple	80
	230

DAY 13 *(cont'd.)*

Lunch

1 small tomato, cut in wedges	30
Salad made of:	
½ 6½-oz. can water-packed tuna	110
½ green pepper, diced	10
1 T. diet mayonnaise	40
dash dry mustard	0
dash paprika	0
2 whole wheat melba toast	30
1 medium peach	40
	260

Dinner

6 oz. (raw weight) flounder or sole, baked or broiled	150
3 oz. green beans with	50
1 tsp. margarine or butter	35
1 small sweet potato baked with	140
1 tsp. butter or margarine	35
½ cantaloupe	35
	415

Snack

1 medium apple	80
	985

Helpful Hints for Day #13

- If poached eggs can't be served immediately, put them in cool water and when you're ready to serve, reheat them gently in hot, salted water.
- Paprika will keep its color and flavor longer if it is stored in the refrigerator.
- Bake sweet potatoes or yams in their skins. When done, cover with a damp cloth. Allow to steam for a few minutes and the skins will peel off easily.

Brunch

Omelet made with:	
1 whole egg and 1 egg white	90
1 T. Parmesan cheese	25
½ green pepper, chopped	10
2 oz. mushrooms, sliced	15
1 oz. Canadian bacon, diced	45
2 slices whole wheat toast	80
with 2 T. unsweetened applesauce and cinnamon	15
½ grapefruit	40
	320

Dinner

5 oz. (raw weight) pork steak, broiled	300
1 C. broccoli (4 spears), steamed	40
with 1 tsp. butter or margarine	35
dash lemon	0
½ C. egg noodles with	100
½ tsp. margarine or butter	35
½ tsp. chives	0
½ cantaloupe with	70
2 oz. vanilla yogurt	50
	630

Snack

1 medium apple	80
	1030

Helpful Hints for Day #14

- You might want to make your own applesauce for the diet.
  After peeling two apples, use a hand grater to slice them into a
  pot containing one-half cup water. Cover and simmer until the
  apples are tender. Then, using a wire whisk, blend the apples to
  the correct consistency.
- Broccoli stems can be cooked in the same length of time as the
  flowerets if you make "X" incisions from top to bottom along the
  stem. Cook the dark green leaves, too: They are extremely
  nutritious.

Chapter 11

Now That You're Ready to Choose Your Own Menus . . .

I know that you're nervous. You're more comfortable with structure, but you've got to learn how to eat like a normal person, and you might as well start now. So you're going to find out how to construct your own diet, which, when you think about it, makes the most sense. If *you* select it, you'll be less likely to rebel against it.

The basic system that follows was developed by many professional health organizations such as the American Dietetic Association. It's especially designed to be used as a life-long plan, and our nutritionist modified it to coordinate with your exercise program and take advantage of the latest information in the field of obesity.

The best part about it is that you'll be eating normal—not diet—foods, which is appropriate if you're going to live the rest of your life like a normal, fit person. This also makes it easy to eat out and cook at home, but it does require a little planning ahead.

Remember: As you lose weight, you must add calories in order to prevent your metabolism from slowing down. You may want some advice as to how you do this. Obviously, you don't just add a scoop of ice cream for each 200-calorie increase you're allowed. For guidance, you can use the chart coming up: Food Groups According to Calorie Value. (Remember also, if you gain a pound or two, cut back to 400 calories until you're at goal. The system that follows can be adapted for this purpose, too.)

Say you're planning a 1200-calorie day. As you read down the column, you see you can have 1 milk, 1 fruit, 2 bread, 2 meat, and 1 fat serving for breakfast, and so on for lunch. The servings come from the lists of Food Groups that follow. In the sample below, I'm going to list calories, but there's actually an easy trick to this. If you follow the food groups, the calories, proteins, carbohydrates, fat, vitamins, and minerals will *automatically* equal up to a balanced diet.

SAMPLE 1200-CALORIE DIET

Food Group	Menu Item	Calorie Count
Breakfast		
1 Milk + 1 Fat	1 C. low-fat yogurt	125
1 Fruit	¾ C. strawberries	40
1 Starch	½ English muffin	70
2 Meat (includes 1 Fat)	2 oz. skim mozzarella	140
Misc./Unlimited	Black coffee	0
		350
Lunch		
1 Free Vegetable	Lettuce	0
2 Meat (low fat)	2 oz. boiled shrimp	110
1 Fat	2 tsp. low-calorie mayonnaise	45
2 Starch	2 slices whole wheat bread	140
1 Fruit	2 medium plums	40
Misc./Unlimited	1 diet soda (restrict to 2 daily)	0
		335
Dinner		
1 Vegetable	½ C. spinach and mushroom salad	25
2 Fat	2 T. oil	90
Free	Vinegar	0
2 Lowfat Meat	Broiled chicken	110
2 Starch	1 small sweet potato	140
1 Fruit	½ grapefruit	40
		405
Snack		
1 Milk	½ C. skim milk	80
1 Fruit	1 peach	40
		120

As you get familiar with the list of Food Groups that follow, you'll soon know which foods are lowest in fat, which are similar in nutritional content, and which can be eaten in any amounts. All of the following Food Group lists contain foods that are approximately equal in protein, carbohydrate, and fat—plus vitamins and minerals.

If you are going out for a special dinner, or if you plan to combine two meals such as brunch, you can "borrow" exchanges from another meal. As a rule, though, you are advised to eat three regular meals plus a fourth light meal made up of a milk and fruit exchange.

What the Food Groups Consist Of

What follows is some of my favorite reading matter—lists of foods. Since the lists are meant to help guide you until you're living like a normal person, many nondiet foods do appear. Of course, it would be impossible to list every food you're likely to eat, but these lists should help guide your selections until you're stabilized at your goal weight.

Normal, fit people don't consult charts when they eat, and neither will you eventually. I hope by the time you feel comfortable without instructions, you will have absorbed the basic principles of sound eating and they'll be second nature.

One final comment about the lists that follow: Don't obsess. The calorie counts are meant to be guidelines. If you notice a ten-calorie discrepancy between one calorie counter and another, don't be concerned. I can assure you that such a discrepancy won't make a significant difference in your weight loss.

FOOD GROUPS ACCORDING TO CALORIC INTAKE

Food Group	1000 Calories	1200 Calories	1400 Calories	1600 Calories	1800 Calories	2000 Calories
Breakfast						
Milk	1	1	1	1	1	1
Fruit	1	1	1	1	1	1
Starch	1	1	2	3	3	3
Meat*	2	2	2	2	2	2
Fat	1	1	1	1	2	2
Lunch						
Free veg.	any	any	any	any	any	any
Fruit	1	1	2	2	3	3
Starch	2	2	2	2	3	3
Meat*	2	2	2	3	3	3
Fat	1	1	2	2	2	3
Dinner						
Milk	0	0	0	0	0	1
Vegetable	1	1	1	1	2	2
Fruit	1	1	2	2	2	2
Starch	1	2	2	2	3	3
Meat*	2	2	2	3	3	3
Fat	1	2	2	2	2	3
Snack						
Milk	0	1	1	1	1	1
Fruit	1	1	1	1	1	1
Summary						
Milk	1	2	2	2	2	3
Fruit	4	4	6	6	6	6
Starch	4	5	6	7	9	9
Meat	6	6	6	8	8	8
Vegetable	2	2	2	2	3	3
Fat	3	4	4	5	6	8

*Use the low-fat meat at least two out of three times daily. This group is lowest in cholesterol as well as fat and calories.

Milk Group

Per serving: 12 grams of carbohydrate, 8 grams of protein, a trace of fat, and 80 calories. Milk products are a major source of calcium, a good source of phosphorus, protein, some B vitamins, vitamins A and D, and some magnesium.

Nonfat

skim or nonfat milk	1 C.
canned evaporated skim milk	½ C.
powdered nonfat dry milk (before adding liquid)	⅓ C.
plain yogurt made from skim milk	1 C.

Low fat*

low-fat milk, 98% fat free	1 C.
low-fat buttermilk	1 C.
plain yogurt made from low-fat milk	1 C.

Full fat†

whole milk	½ C.
goat's milk	½ C.
canned evaporated whole milk	¼ C.
powdered dry milk (before adding liquid)	⅙ C.
plain yogurt made from whole milk	½ C.

Fruit Group

Per serving: 10 grams of carbohydrate and 40 calories. Fruits contain a variety of vitamins and minerals, and are a good source of fiber. Citrus fruits are the best source of vitamin C.

Berries

blackberries	½ C.
blueberries	½ C.
boysenberries	½ C.
cranberries	1 C.
raspberries	½ C.
strawberries	¾ C.

---

*For each serving you select from this group, omit 1 FAT serving from your day's total.

†For each serving you select from this group, omit 2 FAT servings from your day's total.

Fruit Group (cont'd.)

Citrus Fruits

grapefruit	½
orange	½ small
tangelo	1 medium
tangerine	1 medium

Dried Fruits

apricots	4 halves
dates	2 medium
figs	1 medium
peaches	2 halves
pears	2 halves
prunes	2 medium
raisins	2 tsp.

Fruit Juices

apple	⅓ C.
cider	⅓ C.
cranberry	¼ C.
grape	¼ C.
grapefruit	½ C.
nectar	⅓ C.
orange	½ C.
papaya	⅓ C.
pineapple	⅓ C.
prune	¼ C.

Melons

cantaloupe	¼
honeydew	⅛
watermelon	1 C. diced (approx. ½ center slice)

Other Fruits

apple	½ small
applesauce	½ C.
apricots	2 medium
banana	½ small
cherries	10 large

Fruit Group (cont'd.)

grapes	12
kiwi fruit	1 medium
kumquat	2 large
mango	½ small
nectarine	1 small
papaw	1 large
papaya	⅓ medium *or* ½ small *or* ¾ C.
peach	1 medium
pear	1 medium
persimmon	1 medium
pineapple	1 round center slice *or* ½ C.
plums	2 medium
plantain	⅓ small
pomegranate	½ large
quince	⅓ C.

Starch Group

Per serving: 15 grams of carbohydrate, 2 grams of protein, and 70 calories. Whole grain and enriched breads and cereals, along with dried beans and peas, are sources of iron and thiamin. Whole grain products contain more fiber than those made from refined flours. Folacin and potassium are found in many starchy vegetables.

Breads

bagel	½ small
bread (loaf, average size slice)	1 slice
French, Italian, pumpernickel, raisin, rye, white, whole wheat	
biscuit, 2″ diameter*	1
breadcrumbs, dry	3 T.
cornbread, 2″ × 2″ × 1″*	1
English muffin	½
hamburger bun	½
hot dog roll	½

---

*Omit 1 FAT serving.

Breads *(cont'd.)*

muffin, 2″ diameter*	1
pancake, 5″ × ½″*	1
pizza crust	⅛ medium pie
roll, plain	1 small
taco shell	1
tortilla, 6″ diameter	1
waffle, 5″ × ½″*	1
wheat, thin sliced	2 slices

Cereals

barley	1½ T.
bran, unprocessed	¼ C.
bulgur, cooked	½ C.
cereal, cooked	½ C.
cereal, dry:	
All Bran	½ C.
Bran Chex	½ C.
Bran Flakes	¾ C.
Cheerios	¾ C.
Corn Chex	¾ C.
Corn Flakes	¾ C.
Grapenuts	¼ C.
Life	½ C.
Oat Flakes	⅓ C.
Product 19	¾ C.
Puffed Rice	1½ C.
Puffed Wheat	1½ C.
Raisin Bran	½ C.
Rice Chex	¾ C.
Rice Krispies	¾ C.
Shredded Wheat	½ C.
Special K	1 C.
Total	¾ C.
Wheat Chex	½ C.
Wheat Flakes	¾ C.
Wheaties	¾ C.
Chow Mein noodles*	½ C.

*Omit 1 FAT serving.

Cereals *(cont'd.)*

cornmeal, dry	2 T.
flour	2½ T.
grits, cooked	½ C.
kasha, dry (buckwheat groats)	2 T.
pasta, cooked	½ C.
popcorn (popped without added fat)	3 C.
rice or barley, cooked	½ C.
wheat germ, plain	¼ C.

Crackers

arrowroot	3
butter type, round*	5
graham 2½" square	2
matzoth, 4" × 6"	½
melba toast	4
oyster crackers	20
pretzels, 3⅛" long × ⅛" diameter,	25
small twisted	6
rye waffers, 2" × 3½"	3
saltines	6
soda crackers, 2½" square	4
wheat wafers, 2" square	3

Beans

baked beans (without added fat)	¼ C.
dried beans, cooked—red, soy, white,	
black-eyed, cow, split, lentils	½

Starchy Vegetables

corn	⅓ C.
corn on the cob, 6" ear	½
lima beans	½ C.
mixed (carrots, corn, lima, peas)	½ C.
parsnips	½ C.
peas, green	½ C.
potato, white	1 small

---

*Omit 1 FAT serving.

Starchy Vegetables *(cont'd.)*

potato, white mashed	½ C.
pumpkin	1 C.
sweet potato or yam	½ small *or* ¼ C.
winter squash	½ C.
acorn	
butternut	
banana	

Prepared Foods

angel food cake	1 small slice, *or* 1½″ cube
chips, potato or corn†	15
crepe, 6″ diameter*	1
ice milk	½ C.
potatoes, french fried*	8
sherbet, fruit ice	½ C.

Meat Group

All of these foods are excellent sources of protein and many are good sources of iron, zinc, vitamin B_{12}, and other B vitamins. Try to limit your intake of red meat, increasing instead poultry and fish. The latter contain smaller amounts of cholesterol. Remember that the following three meat groups are slightly different and that at least 2 of your 3 daily meat *portions* (breakfast, lunch, and dinner) should come from the low fat, group A meats.

All canned fish should be packed in water. Meats should be trimmed of all visible fat. Have beef trimmed before being ground. Cook without added fat.

Low Fat

Each serving contains 7 grams of protein, 3 grams of fat, and 55 calories.

---

*Omit 1 FAT serving.
†Omit 2 FAT servings.

Low Fat *(cont'd.)*

Beef

chuck (not ground)	1 oz.
dried beef	1 oz.
flank steak (sirloin, tenderloin)	1 oz.
plate skirt steak	1 oz.
round (not ground)	1 oz.
tripe	1 oz.

Cheese

cottage, dry or low-fat	¼ C.
ricotta, part skim	1 oz.
St. Otho Swiss	1 oz.
low-fat cheeses, less than 5% butterfat	3 T.

Fish

any, fresh or frozen	1 oz.
fish or shellfish, canned	¼ C.
sardines, drained	3 medium
shellfish, fresh or frozen	1 oz.

Frog legs 1 oz.

Lamb

all cuts except breast and ground	1 oz.

Pork

leg	1 oz.
fresh or smoked ham, all cuts	1 oz.

Poultry (without skin)

chicken	1 oz.
hen	1 oz.
pheasant	1 oz.
turkey	1 oz.

Rabbit 1 oz.

Tofu (soybean curd) 2½ oz.

Veal

all cuts except breast and ground	1 oz.

Venison 1 oz.

Medium Fat

Each serving contains 7 grams of protein, 5 grams of fat, and 75 calories.

Beef

corned beef (canned)	1 oz.
porterhouse	1 oz.
rib-eye	1 oz.
T-bone	1 oz.
tongue	1 oz.
toploin	1 oz.

Cheese

cottage, creamed	1/4 C.
farmer's	1 oz.
Neufchâtel	1 oz.
processed spread	1 oz.
skim American	1 oz.
skim mozzarella	1 oz.

Eggs 1

Organ meats

heart	1 oz.
kidney	1 oz.
liver	1 oz.
sweetbreads	1 oz.

Pork

Canadian bacon	1 oz.
ham (boiled, canned, country-style)	1 oz.
loin (all chops, blade roast, rib half or whole, sirloin cutlets or ribs, toploin roast)	1 oz.
shoulder arm picnic	1 oz.
smoked pork shoulder (picnic, roll)	1 oz.

High Fat*

Each serving contains 7 grams of protein, 8 grams of fat, and 100 calories.

Beef
brisket	1 oz.
ground beef, commercial	1 oz.

Cheese
American	1 oz.
blue—Roquefort	1 oz.
brick	1 oz.
Camembert	1 oz.
cheddar	1 oz.
colby	1 oz.
limburger	1 oz.
Parmesan	1 oz.
processed products	1 oz.
provolone	1 oz.
Romano	1 oz.
Swiss	1 oz.

Cold cuts	1 oz.
Hot dog	1 oz.

Lamb
breast, ground	1 oz.

Peanut butter	1½ T.

Pork
deviled ham	1 oz.
loin (back ribs, country pork)	1 oz.
spareribs	1 oz.

Poultry
capon	1 oz.
duck (domestic)	1 oz.
goose	1 oz.

Sausage	1 oz.

*Omit 1 FAT serving for each of the following items.

High Fat *(cont'd.)*
Veal
    breast, ground   1 oz.

Vegetable Group*

Per serving: 5 grams of carbohydrate, 2 grams of protein, and 25 calories.

Dark green and deep yellow vegetables are terrific sources of vitamin A. Use different vegetables each day to get vitamin C, folacin, and B_6. All vegetables contain fiber.

Free: Eat these as you desire.

chicory	all types of lettuce
Chinese cabbage	parsley
endive	radishes
escarole	

Restricted: One serving equals ½ cup or value specified.

alfalfa sprouts	greens:
artichoke (1 medium)	beet
asparagus	chard
bamboo shoots	collards
bean sprouts	dandelion
beans, green or wax	kale
beets	mustard
broccoli	spinach
brussels sprouts	turnip
cabbage	leeks
carrots (½ cup *or* 1 medium)	mushrooms
cauliflower	okra (8–9 pods)
celery	onions
Chinese pea pods	pepper, green and red
cucumber	pimentos
eggplant	rhubarb

---

*Starchy vegetables are included in the Starch Group.

Vegetable Group (cont'd.)

rutabagas
sauerkraut
squash:
    patty pan
    scallop
    summer
    zucchini

tomato juice
tomatoes
turnips
vegetable juice cocktail
water chestnuts

Fat Group

Per serving: 5 grams of fat and 45 calories. Since these are concentrated sources of calories, they must be measured especially carefully. Try to use fats or vegetable rather than animal origin, because they are lower in saturated fat and higher in unsaturated fat. (See Second Helpings for an explanation.)

avocado, 4″	⅛
bacon	1 strip
bacon fat	1 tsp.
butter	1½ tsp. *or* 1 pat
chocolate, unsweetened	2 tsp. *or* ⅓ oz.
coconut, dried	2 T.
coconut milk	4 tsp.
cocoa, dry powder	3 T.
cream:	
half and half	3 T.
heavy	1 T.
heavy, whipped	2 T.
light	2 T.
nondairy	2 T.
sour	2 T.
cream cheese	1 T.
lard	1 tsp.
margarine	1½ tsp.
margarine, low calorie	2 tsp.
mayonnaise	1 tsp.
mayonnaise, low calorie	2 tsp.

Fat Group (cont'd.)
nuts:

almonds	10 whole
macadamia	3
peanuts	20 whole
pecans, large	2
pistachios	20
other	6
oil	1 tsp.
olives	5 small

Salad dressing

blue cheese or Roquefort	2 tsp.
French	1 T.
Italian	2 tsp.
mayonnaise-type	1 T.
Russian	2 tsp.
Thousand Island	2 tsp.
tartar sauce	1 T.

Miscellaneous

Per serving: 0 or neglible calories. Eat as desired (except where noted).

artificial sweetener
bouillon, clear fat-free* *or* low-sodium *or* fat-free brands
club soda* *or* low-sodium *or* fat-free brands
coffee†
gelatin, sugar-free or unflavored
gum, sugar-free
herbs
horseradish
lemon
lime
mineral water

---

*All high in salt. Keep it to one pickle and 2 glasses of any of these drinks daily, unless your doctor advises less.
†High in caffeine (see Second Helpings), so you may want to limit your intake.

Miscellaneous (cont'd.)
mustard (use catsup sparingly)
pickles: dill or sour*
soft drinks, sugar-free*
spices
tea†
vinegar†

Alcohol
Count alcohol as a FAT. The calories in alcohol can be calculated: 0.8 × proof × ounces = calories. Each 45 calories should be counted as 1 FAT serving. Dry wines and light beers are good choices. Liqueurs and sweet mixed drinks contain considerable quantities of sugar and should be avoided.

---

*All high in salt. Keep it to one pickle and 2 glasses of any of these drinks daily, unless your doctor advises less.
†High in caffeine (see Second Helpings), so you may want to limit your intake.

Chapter 12

The Walkout—
Easier Than a Workout

You're probably a little skeptical about this walking business. You've been on a diet before, and I'm sure mine makes sense to you. But *walking*? I bet that secretly you don't believe it will work.

But this is a fact: In a university study, overweight women who made no change in their eating habits but walked at least thirty minutes a day lost an average of twenty-two pounds per year.

Next you're going to be telling me you really need spot-reducing. And I'll tell you there is no such thing. In a study at the University of Massachusetts, twenty-one people involved in a rigorous program of situps were found to have lost a small amount of fat from their middles—but also from their backs and backsides. Exercise doesn't help you lose weight from a specific spot.

Women put on weight in a predetermined fashion: first on the back of the thigh, then the inside, and next, in order, hips, midriff, and upper body (such as arms). Fat will decrease in reverse order from the way it was put on—no matter what specific exercise you do. By working on a specific muscle as you do in a situp, you just develop that muscle and make it larger, while the fat stays on top of it. Only aerobic exercise, which draws fat equally from every part of the body, will help change your shape.

Next you're going to be telling me you already walk a lot. A plump friend of mine from Los Angeles used to tell me that she was a great walker. She came along with me one day—I'd been walking for about four months at the time—and I kept my usual pace, or perhaps even a bit slower. After the walk, we went different ways, and then I called her later in the afternoon to confirm our dinner plans. She had to cancel: She'd taken to her bed with exhaustion.

Let me tell you something. If you really *are* walking a lot, then you don't have a fat problem. If you do, then you only *think* you're walking a lot.

Why walking and not weightlifting. There are two kinds of exercises. One kind, such as weightlifting, sprinting, golf, even calisthenics, is stop-and-start exercising. The other is continuous exercise—such as jogging, dancing, and walking. Exercise in this category is considered "aerobic."

"Aerobic" exercise uses oxygen. During the course of aerobic exercise, your heart beats faster, your lungs expand, and your blood vessels open up in order to carry blood loaded with oxygen to the cells. The more oxygen you use, the more fat gets burned. The most popular aerobic exercises are swimming, bicycling, jumping rope, dancing, jogging, and walking.

What to tell your friends when they recommend jogging. Lots of folks aren't that crazy about the alternatives to walking. I'm not. Take swimming: You have to change out of your clothes into your suit, then back again. It takes up a lot of time. Then you get your hair wet, and either you get one of those short haircuts or you arrive back at your office with a fresh-out-of-the-sauna look. I don't know about you, but I don't think I'm blond or Nordic enough for that. Jumping rope doesn't interest me. I've tried bicycling, but once the snows start, it's out of the question. Besides, once you're on your bike, you're committed to it. Suppose you feel like walking back? I've tried the stationary bicycle, but I feel the way I do when I take gas at the dentist's office: Time is standing still. Dancing is nice, but I remember being asked to sign a medical release when I signed up for class. I think that if you're not in shape, it's just too much. Besides, I know you aren't too anxious to get into a leotard when you feel more like a wreckette than a Rockette.

And then there's jogging. Now, I've tried it, as I mentioned, and I didn't like it. For one thing, I find it aesthetically unappealing to see big women jogging. Besides, I don't think it's natural for human beings. Animals do it, but animals move on all fours.

In fact, I see that scientists have a lot of animals out jogging these days. A bunch of jogging monkeys were used in research to determine if people who exercised would have arteries that were less clogged than those who didn't. There was even a group of "Yucatan mini swine"—that's pigs, to you and me—who were running a hundred miles a week around a San Diego laboratory to prove that exercise could be beneficial even if your arteries were clogged.

(It seems to be; but walking is exercise, too.) I prefer to leave the jogging to animals; they do very well at it.

Jogging can also lead to problems—skeletal injuries, foot problems, organ displacement, stress fractures, sprains, and breaks. Even eye problems, like detached retinas, and ear problems connected with balance are linked to jogging. Moreover, as you get older, the situation gets worse. Your ligaments and tendons lose their flexibility, making it easier to break limbs, dislocate joints, and tear muscles. You might end up a perfect cardiovascular specimen using a cane.

And here's, so to speak, a kick in the teeth: It seems that if you jog without a bra, your breasts can slap against you with as much as seventy pounds of pressure.

It also turns out that walking five miles may take longer than jogging five miles but they both burn off the same number of calories.

Walking definitely works to make you lean and fit. In many ways it seems to be the best exercise you can do. Here are some of the reasons:

1. Walking is easy. I have actually read books that include instructions on how to walk, but almost everyone I've met past the age of about fourteen months seems to have it down pat.
2. Walking is cheap, particularly since you're supposed to be walking too fast to window-shop.
3. You can't hurt yourself. Well, I suppose you could, but why aren't you looking where you're going?
4. You can camouflage yourself. I now believe that thin people probably thought, At least she's trying to do something about herself, but I used to think they considered me a comical sight when I was out exercising. Still, no out-of-shape person likes to draw attention—but you can walk in the middle of crowds.
5. It's efficient. You can transport yourself and exercise yourself at the same time. Look at the fuel you're saving. I was toying with the idea of just throwing away my car keys.
6. You don't have to change clothes to walk, and you won't need a shower and another change to look presentable whenever you get where you're going.

The Walkout—
How to Do It

Frequency

At least five times a week. A 1980 study showed that exercise four and five times a week is three times as effective as exercise three times a week. Exercise once or twice a week is almost useless. *Also, don't skip two days in a row.*

Time of Day

Before a meal or up to one hour after. There is some indication that fat storage pathways are more efficient at night, so it *may* be helpful to exercise then. If you've done your aerobic exercise before eating, you may want to take a little extra, moderate walk directly after eating to take advantage of dietary thermogenesis. (Even if you do your aerobic exercise as much as an hour after a meal, you will still take advantage of dietary thermogenesis.)

Amount

Start at twenty minutes and work up to sixty. Take it slow for the first couple of weeks: Start with twenty minutes per day, then go up to thirty. You're out of shape and I can't promise you this will be fun. It won't be aerobic either, since that requires at least thirty minutes of continuous exercise plus warmup time. Walking during the first two weeks is just meant to get you out the door.

Remember: Walking is not a punishment. It becomes a routine, like brushing your teeth, but, it also becomes a pleasure. You will start looking forward to your walk.

Do not overexert the first few days. You may decide you can do better than you're supposed to. Don't get so carried away that you spend the next couple of days lying in bed with warm towels to recuperate. You've destroyed the whole purpose of the walking, which is that it must be done regularly.

Dr. Joel told me to set aside an hour a day for walking. The hour could *include* ten minutes of warmup and ten of cool down, he said, but I'd be better off doing the warmup in addition to an hour of brisk walking. At the end of this section, you'll find some warmup exercises. As for cooling down, you do that simply by slowing down your pace. When you're walking at top speed, you're using your heart to pump extra blood into your arms and legs. If you stop too abruptly, you may get some cramping.

Not until you've walked quickly, for at least thirty minutes, does fat burning take place. As you know, the body first burns carbohydrates for energy, and only after it uses them up does it go to the fat stores.

Speed

Until you're moving at 70 percent of maximum heart rate. You saw the word percent and figured you weren't going to like this part, right? Numbers are not something I'm fond of, either. They bring up unpleasant associations: how many pounds on the scale, how many inches around my thigh, how many calories in this portion. But please bear with me; I have to talk about numbers here.

Dr. Joel pointed out to me that when he said to walk, he meant *move.* You're not supposed to be window-shopping; you're supposed to be pretending that Norman Bates (from *Psycho*) is after you. Walk with a purpose: You do have one, of course.

The best way to gauge yourself is to take your own pulse.

For the wrist pulse: Press the first two fingers of your right hand (if you're right-handed) across the opposite forearm, about an inch above the wrist. Press hard enough to feel the thumping of the blood but not so hard that you block it off. Time yourself using a clock with a second hand. Count the first beat as zero.

For the neck pulse: This might be easier for you. Place the first three fingers of your hand just below the angle of the jaw. Stretch your neck out, and move your fingers slowly down your neck until you feel the beat. *Do not press*—you're supposed to *feel* the beat, not halt it. Press too hard and you'll cut off the blood vessel.

Do you remember hearing that 72 was the perfect pulse rate? Most Americans' pulses are in the eighties and nineties, but someone in good condition can have a pulse rate of 65 or lower.

How hard you're exercising is determined by how fast your pulse is moving. The rate you strive for is calculated after you've figured out your maximum pulse rate.

To find your maximum pulse rate, subtract your age from the number 220. If you're 40, your maximum rate is 180. (220 − 40 = 180) Of course, you don't exercise to the maximum. Right now I'm sure you couldn't. And if you could, you would pass out fairly soon. Athletes in excellent shape push themselves to about 85 percent and you should strive for about 70 percent.

If your maximum pulse rate is 180, multiply that by 70 percent and you'll see that your exercise rate should be 126. (180 × .70 = 126).

Exercise Heart Rates

Age	Maximum Rate	10-second count (70% of maximum)	Age	Maximum Rate	10-second count (70% of maximum)
18	202	24	45	175	20
19	201	23	46	174	20
20	200	23	47	173	20
21	199	23	48	172	20
22	198	23	49	171	20
23	197	23	50	170	20
24	196	23	51	169	20
25	195	23	52	168	20
26	194	23	53	167	19
27	193	23	54	166	19
28	192	22	55	165	19
29	191	22	56	164	19
30	190	22	57	163	19
31	189	22	58	162	19
32	188	22	59	161	19
33	187	22	60	160	19
34	186	22	61	159	19
35	185	22	62	158	18
36	184	21	63	157	18
37	183	21	64	156	18
39	181	21	66	154	18
40	180	21	67	153	18
41	179	21	68	152	18
42	178	1	69	151	18
43	177	20	70	150	18
44	176	20			

I suggest you find out what your 10-second rate should be (in this case it's 21, since 21 × 6 = 126). This is because while you're out walking and checking your pulse, it's more efficient to stop for only ten seconds rather than a minute. With the following chart, I've spared you the trouble of figuring this out for yourself.

After the first five to ten minutes of exercising, you should get up to 50 percent of maximum rate. The worse shape you're in, the faster it will get there.

I know you'll be tempted to stop much too often to check your pulse, so here's a rule-of-thumb test to see if you've reached your 70 percent of maximum level. If you can carry on a conversation or—just barely—manage to sing out loud, you're probably going along at the right speed.

Just remember: The more you walk, and the faster you walk, the quicker that weight will come off and the faster you'll shape up.

Distance

3¹/₂ or 4 miles per hour is what you're striving for.

The major reason you're walking is to rebuild the lean muscle mass in your body and increase thermogenesis, but remember you're also walking to burn up calories. The way to gauge that is to find out how much ground you've covered.

The figure of calories burned is only an estimate because the number is influenced by several factors including weight, age, sex, general fitness, and the genetic variations between individuals.

Scientists figure out how many calories you burn by measuring how much oxygen you use. If you use one liter of oxygen, you burn 4.82 calories a minute. So if a hundred-pound person uses a third of a liter of oxygen in a minute of dishwashing, she uses up a third of 4.8, or about 1.6 calories per minute.

The more frequently and more deeply you breathe during exercise, the more oxygen you use; and the more oxygen you use, the more calories you burn.

Here's a guide to measure how many calories you're burning an hour. Multiply your weight times the figure below:

If you're walking 2 miles per hour, multiply your weight by 1.30

2¹/₄	1.56
3	1.80
3¹/₄	2.05
4	2.35
4¹/₄	3.10
5	3.85

In other words, if you weigh 200 and you're going 2 miles per hour, you're burning 260 calories (1.30 × 260).

How fast you go is partly determined by the length of your legs, too: A short-legged person might find a pace of 20 minutes per mile or 3 miles per hour moderate and 15 minutes per mile or 4 miles per hour fast, while a taller person might manage a 17-minute mile moving moderately and an 11–12-minute mile moving quickly.

That's it. That's all you have to know. Just get out there and start walking.

Warmup Exercises

I'm suggesting a few, but there are quite a number of variations that would be acceptable. Perhaps you even have an old exercise book lying around the house that you always meant to do something about. Use it. Or follow these:

Loosening Up

1. Stand tall, with your feet about twelve inches apart. Breathe deeply in and out. Ten times in all.
2. Stand tall. Stick arms straight out. Make ten pumpkin-sized circles forward, then ten in reverse. Repeat.
3. Stand tall. Close eyes, relax jaw, drop your head forward. Rotate your head ten times clockwise, then ten times counterclockwise.
4. Stand tall. Rotate shoulders forward ten times, then backward ten times.

Stretching

1. Toes. Sit on floor with legs in front of you straight out. Keep heels on the floor. Point your toes all the way forward and hold for a count of ten, then point your toes toward your body, hold for a count of ten. Fifteen times for each foot.
2. Ankles. Remain sitting, with legs straight out. Lift your foot and rotate your ankle, making large circles ten times in one direction, then ten in reverse direction. Repeat with other foot.
3. Feet. Sit on floor crosslegged, left foot on top of right thigh. Grab the foot with both hands, the sole in the left hand, the top with the right hand. Don't move your leg or your knee; just bend the ankle. Then twist your foot so that the sole points upward and you feel a pull. Hold for a count of ten. Repeat with other foot.
4. Calves. Stand about arm's length from a wall. Stretch one leg out behind you, keeping the knee straight. Slightly bend the knee of the forward leg. Keeping both heels on the floor, lean in against the wall until you feel a pull. Hold for a count of fifteen. Repeat with other leg. Do this eight times with each leg.

5. **Front of thigh.** Stand. Hold your right heel in your right hand and pull gently. If you can, pull the foot up to touch your hip. Hold for a count of ten. Repeat with other leg. Five times for each leg.
6. **Back of thigh.** Put your right foot on a table about three feet high. Now bend over and reach for your left toes with both hands. Keep legs and back straight. Feel the pull in the back of your thighs and lower back. Hold for a count of ten. Repeat with other leg. Ten times for each leg.
7. **Whole body.** Put your feet two feet apart and bend forward, stretching from lower back. Grab your right ankle with both hands and bring your face down to your knee. Hold for a count of ten. Repeat with other leg. Five times for each leg.

Weather or Not

Rain

You wake up, take a look out the window, and see it's raining. You think, Great! At least I don't have to do that walking stuff today. You're wrong. Today is a day like any other. Get out there. Put on your raincoat and go through that front door. Now I'm not suggesting you go out into a tornado, but a little rain never hurt anyone. If you get yourself a good slicker and some comfortable boots, the rain won't even bother you. Still, if you can't stand the sound of mud oozing underfoot, let me remind you that there are some places you can walk indoors.

- Shopping malls. Almost every city has one. Just don't stop where they're selling food. You're not supposed to stop while you're walking anyway. You might plan to have your fourth meal and a cup of black coffee when the hour's over.
- Indoor tracks. You'd be surprised at how many Y's and schools have tracks available for public use. Let your fingers do the walking to locate a place where your legs can do the walking.
- Airports. I don't mean the runway. I mean inside. Airports in major cities are huge. Going from one end to the other is a great way to kill time and keep you out of the cocktail lounge.
- Museums. Walk through at a brisk pace. Don't feel strange. Just pretend you're looking for someone. This may prove to be a

problem if it rains for several days on end or if you live in Puget Sound, where I understand it never *stops* raining. The guards become suspicious. On the other hand, you might get a reputation as a real art lover. Make sure that during your cool down, when you're going a little more slowly, you actually do look at what's hanging on the walls. Someone might ask you about the current show.

One place I wouldn't suggest you do your walking: a super-market.

You might want some suggestions for equipment:

- Slicker. Keep one of those foldup ones with you at all times. Get something with a hood. I don't know about you, but I never feel as if I can really *move* with an umbrella.
- Boots. Make sure they're waterproof. Wet feet cause blisters, aside from feeling awful.

Keep thinking how great the rain is for your skin. English beauties, who are famous for their clear complexions, get them from walking through the mists on the moors.

Cold

Don't tell me you can't walk in the cold. I do, and I live in Minneapolis, where even the ground hogs don't come out in February. Get into your coat and your mittens and remind yourself how cute you look when your face is flushed from the cold.

- Bonus: Moderately overweight people who do aerobic exercise in cold weather burn extra fat.
- Walk into the wind (it's colder) at the beginning of your walk, and away from it as you return.
- Skin freezes at 25° F. and below. You might want to consider wearing a ski mask if it's really frigid out.
- Wear a hat. You lose a great deal of your body heat through your head.
- Your battery-operated cassette player may go on the fritz in the cold, since the lower temperature slows down the chemical action used to make electricity. Keep it under heavy clothes and close to your body. Once you're inside, the power will return to normal.

116

Hot Weather

- A lightweight hat soaked in water and squeezed dry might help keep you cool.
- Drink extra water. This not only prevents heat exhaustion but if you become dehydrated, your body confuses thirst and hunger and you become ravenous.
- If you have muscle cramps in your legs, that may indicate that you need more potassium—which is lost, together with sodium, when you sweat. Drink eight ounces of skim milk; eat a fruit that's high in potassium, such as melons, bananas, oranges, and apricots, or choose a potato at dinner.

Shoes

I have bought many pairs of walking shoes, but not until 1982 did I actually wear out a pair. I used to think of them as cruel shoes, but now I don't go anywhere without them. If I go to a formal I have them in a bag in my car. A few words about shoes:

- Use running shoes for walking. Nylon uppers are good for hot weather because they allow circulation; and leather uppers are good in rainy and snowy weather. They keep out wetness, which causes blisters.
- Remove scuffs on white leather uppers with typewriter correction fluid.
- When new ones are stiff, bend them at the ball of the foot, then tape them in that position and leave that way overnight.
- If nylon uppers on your shoes get wet, stuff them with newspapers and let dry (away from heat and direct sunlight at room temperature).

... And Socks

- Wear two pair of thin socks rather than one pair of thick ones to keep in the heat and reduce the chance of getting a blister. (If you do get one, cut a piece of foam into a square, cut a hole in the foam, and tape it over the blister.)
- Buy a pair of silk socks to put under your other ones. They're terrific for keeping the heat in.

Equipment

- One other piece of equipment you might enjoy: a pedometer.
- For about $70 you might treat yourself to a Japanese-made Jogger Mate Pulse Meter. About the size of a business card, it's a little boxlike gizmo into which you insert your pinky. A moving needle registers your pulse.
- Major splurge: a treadmill. I have one and it's the greatest. (Now I know somebody is going to ask how come I hate stationary bicycles and love my treadmill. On both of them, you're going nowhere; but on a stationary bicycle you're going there faster. What's the rush?)

How to Get Yourself Going: Buy a Portable Cassette Player You Can Wear on Your Waist

There's nothing like music with a beat to get you going. I started off with "Sixteen Tons" and now I'm ready to move to "The Flight of the Bumblebee." You can listen to your favorite music, of course, but there are other special things you can do with your player and headphones:

- Tape the soap operas while you're doing something else around the house, then catch up with "Days of Our Lives" or "The Young and the Restless" while you're out walking the next day. You may have to use your imagination during some of the quiet spots, but that might be a plus.
- Buy a tape that helps you learn a foreign language.
- Instead of writing a letter to someone, tape your message while you walk, and ask for a taped letter in reply.
- Tape a speech you have to give and play it back so you can memorize it.
- While your head is clear, record a list of all the things you have to accomplish—short-term or long-term.
- Learn the lyrics to songs you always wanted to be able to sing along with.
- Listen to a tape recording of a play instead of music for a change. You can probably borrow one from your library.

118

I'd Rather Walk Alone

You're going to read here and there about how you should organize groups of friends, neighbors, and colleagues to walk with you. I think this is a big bunch of baloney. The first rainy day that comes along, they'll all cop out on you. My friends did. They didn't have my fat problem, and so they didn't have the motivation that I did—and you will.

I know sometimes you'll find it difficult to keep on walking, but remember that you have to work very hard to be normal again. One of my good friends, a woman who always has had a terrific body, promised to come along with me one day and sure enough, the weather was rotten and she decided to stay home. So there I was with my parka on, and my hat and my ear muffs and my gloves, pushing along and feeling really sorry for myself. Why me? I was thinking. Why do I have to work this hard? Of course, I was sure I was the only one suffering the way I was. Then I got out to the lake and there were dozens of people out there doing the same thing I was, either to get in shape or stay in shape. (If you have a vengeful streak, maybe it will make you feel better to think that someday it'll catch up with them. The friends sitting home will be huffing and puffing at some future date to work off those extra pounds they're putting on now.)

Enjoy being out there and being by yourself. At least you don't have to listen to Joe Blow's office politics or the marital saga of Sally Smith.

Another bonus: the sound of silence. If you've spent most of your life trying to tune out the din of an office or assorted kids, pets, and other loved ones, you might find you're crazy about being alone with yourself. Walking gives you some time alone that you'd probably otherwise find impossible to get. If you get too lonely, just turn on your portable cassette player and let Willie Nelson romance you.

Walking Not Only Makes You Fit and Lean, but Also

- Improves your circulation. Your hands and feet won't get as cold as they used to.
- Reduces your chances of getting osteoporosis, a bone disease

not uncommon in older women, since increased strength, fitness, and activity help prevent weak bones.

- Lessens the chance of hardening of the arteries by increasing HDL cholesterol, a blood protein that transports the other kind of cholesterol out of the artery walls. That makes you less susceptible to stroke and heart attack in later middle age and old age.
- Stimulates you to secrete sleep-inducing endorphins. You'll have the soundest sleep you've ever had. Now I find I don't sleep unless I've walked. So I've got two motivators: staying fit and sleeping. Otherwise I might be up all night eating.
- Helps prevent the kind of diabetes that's common in middle age.
- Improves your posture, which results in fewer back pains, aching legs, and varicose veins and also builds abdominal muscles.
- Lets you walk your problems away. You may not get rid of them, but you'll sure get the tension out of your system.

Chapter 13

Mary Ellen's Forty-four Best Diet Tips

1. Make a Doctor's Appointment and Keep It
You've read this warning in every diet book you've ever read.

WARNING
Do not embark on this or any other
diet program without first
consulting your physician.

But you didn't, did you? You knew if you marched in there with that
cockamamie diet you last went on your doctor would have laughed
you right out of the office. Well, I'm telling you to see your doctor,
and I mean it. I'm not saying it as a disclaimer so that if something
goes wrong, I won't get in hot water. I'm saying it so something goes
right. If you're in the same shape as I was before I went to Dr. Joel,
you're probably long overdue for a checkup anyway. Just make sure
the doctor is someone you can trust. And who knows? Maybe you'll
be one of the lucky ones and it will turn out your weight problem is a
thyroid condition after all.

2. Quit Procrastinating
I know all the excuses. I've used them myself. I once put
off starting my next diet until the coming of Halley's
Comet. As you may recall, Halley's Comet comes around once in
every seventy-six years and it had been seen the day before I made
my vow. There is no rule that you have to wait until Monday to start
a diet, or until after the holidays: It won't be a less joyful Christmas
if you're not stuffing yourself along with the goose. If you're the way
I was, when you're not dieting, you're gaining. The longer you put

the diet off, the fatter you're going to be when you finally start it. So pick up the phone and make a doctor's appointment *now*, and before you get there finish this book and start planning your walking schedule. (You can buy your walking shoes and diet groceries on the way home from the doctor's office.)

3. *Forget Being a Big Beautiful Doll Unless You Are One*

You've seen the models in the large-size clothing catalogs. They weigh two hundred pounds and more, their bodies are firm as the Rock of Gibraltar, and they look great. But I don't think the average shopper in Queen Bee or Elegant X or those other places that cater to larger women is cover girl material. If I had looked like a BBD, I'd have been proud; but the only modeling agency that would have hired me at 208 was an outfit called Funny Face. If you're big and beautiful, all you have to do is start looking for larger men to look good next to. But I don't think there are too many BBG's (Big Beautiful Guys) out there either.

4. *Eat Meals on Regular-Size Plates*

I don't believe in the school of thought that says you should put your food on doll plates so you think there's more of it. You'd better learn what six ounces of chicken looks like so you can gauge what you're eating anywhere. And that advice about always leaving something on your plate leaves me cold, too. If you're not supposed to be eating it, what's it doing on your plate anyway?

5. *Write Down Whatever You Eat*

And I mean *everything*. The dab of butter here, the bite of apple there. All that stuff that adds up to a few billion calories if you don't keep track. At the end of Part Three, Second Helpings, there's a sample diary page. Make yourself a few photocopies and tuck them in your bag along with a pencil. Be as faithful in keeping a record as you were with your first diary.

6. *If You're Having a Craving, Wait Twenty Minutes Before You Give In*

There it is: That piece of cake left over from your son's birthday party. You want it, don't you? Stop. First drink a glass of water, then find something else to do for twenty minutes. Walk. Read a book. Call an old boyfriend. Nine out of ten times, the urge will have passed. Whatever was luring you with its siren call won't seem too appealing after you've delayed the gratification.

. . . And if you eat it after all, then go out and walk for fifteen minutes.

So you ate it. I hope it tasted good. Now forget it, stop guilt-tripping, and leave the house. Take a fifteen-minute bonus walk. You just turned a negative situation into a positive one. As you walk, remind yourself, "I'll do better next time."

7. To Err Is Human, to Binge Divine

Let's face it. You're going to cheat once in a while. I did, and that's normal. I must tell you it got easier to stay on the program once I started getting results; also, after a while I lost my desire for some of the junk that had tempted me in the past. But there were occasions when I went out to dinner or to a party and went a little overboard. In some cases, I jumped ship entirely. The next morning, I'd get up, and instead of starting the day with a pint of Haagen-Dazs, I'd eat my normal breakfast, do my walking, and just get back with the program. (I didn't cut back because I slipped, either.) Most diets fail because someone says, "I ate too much last night; I've ruined everything anyway."

8. Eat Four Times a Day

I thought I was doing myself a favor when I skipped breakfast. If I wasn't hungry, why should I eat? I always viewed breakfast as extra, useless calories. I often skipped lunch, too. By dinnertime, I wanted something really substantial, like a tree. I started at six o'clock and kept on going, with occasional breaks, until midnight. Now I know it's important to eat regularly. You get less hungry, so you don't gorge. Besides, when you eat, you start dietary thermogenesis, the process in which your body burns extra calories just in the act of processing foods. When you don't eat, you miss out on this process and reduce your metabolism rate, too. It may be called *fasting*, but it actually slows you down.

9. Eating Between Meals

Let's be honest. There isn't a Baggie in the world big enough to carry around all the food you really want. When you're eating a carrot stick, you don't want a carrot stick. You want a nice big hunk of chocolate cake.

Why should I tell you to carry an apple around if you get hungry between meals? Do I think you're going to say, "What a great idea! I'll have an apple instead of a candy bar"? If you were the kind of person who chooses apples between meals, you wouldn't be overweight in the first place.

All you're doing with the carrot and the celery and the apples is substituting one kind of eating for another. And what you should be doing is training yourself to eat only at meals. If you're following the program properly, you shouldn't be hungry between meals anyway.

10. Don't Eat to Pep Yourself Up

Most of us think if we eat a little something, we'll feel better. If we're feeling blah, food will give us instant energy. Think about it. "Energetic" is not a word often applied to people who are eating all the time. Eating is not a cure-all.

If you're feeling dizzy and tired, get out of the kitchen and into bed so you don't fall over the stove or into the refrigerator and hurt yourself. I'm joking, but the point is, if you're eating properly, you won't get dizzy and tired in the first place. Next time you're about to make a little excursion into the fridge, stop for a moment and ask if you're experiencing true hunger.

Do you just want junk food? Have you had a real meal within the past two hours? Has something upset you or made you happy? What you're feeling isn't hunger.

Or have you skipped a meal? Has it been four hours since you've eaten? Would you be satisfied with a nutritious meal instead of junk food? Is your stomach growling? Do you feel really empty? Any of these symptoms means you're feeling true hunger, and it's time for a meal.

11. Put Your Fork Down Between Bites

Put your spoon and knife down, too. Straws aren't allowed either. Have a little conversation during the meal. Don't dive into your food. Watch thin people eat. They sometimes hold something on their fork and forget about it while they talk. Bet you never did that.

Did you know that speed eaters can consume three courses in twenty gulps? Twenty dips and it's all over. They're like high-powered vacuum cleaners. You have to learn to be a carpet sweeper.

Here's how you do it. For lunch, plan to eat for thirty minutes. For dinner, plan on thirty to forty-five. Put the fork down with each bite. Chew each mouthful eight to ten times. Swallow and count four seconds before you put the fork back in your food. Do this for two days.

This is very difficult to do. I want you to know that. These meals will not go down in history as among the best you have ever eaten. In fact, the food may seem repulsive to you. That's not the point. What this is intended to do—and it will—is slow you down. It works. After a couple of days, you'll slow down automatically. You won't be counting the minutes every time you have a meal.

12. Eat at the Table

Food has always been my friend. In fact, I rarely went anywhere without it. It's even been with me in the bathroom: olive oil on my scalp, egg yolks and mayonnaise on my face, and potato chips on my lips. The oil was to restore the natural luster of my hair, and I used the egg yolks and mayo for a facial mask. The potato chips weren't part of the beauty treatment. They were just keeping me company.

My friend Gail's family gathers around the portable dishwasher, which serves as a smorgasbord table, to snack between meals. Their theory is that if you eat standing up, it doesn't count. It does, of course. Remember: Elephants eat standing up.

You bought your kitchen or dining room table to have your meals there—not just to cut out patterns on or do your kids' homework at. Try using it for its original purpose again. If you know you have to be sitting down to have a meal, you're not going to sneak in calories on the run.

13. Don't Do Anything Else While You Eat

Remember the guy who couldn't walk and chew gum at the same time? He got to be President. Take a leaf from his book, and when you're chewing, don't do anything else. Eating is a legitimate activity. It deserves its own slot in your schedule. Enjoy your food. Don't grab it on the run. Don't shovel it down while you're reading the latest Mitchener novel. Don't fork it in while you're watching TV; during those suspenseful shows, it can really go down fast. When you concentrate on something else, you forget you're eating; and when you forget you're eating, you eat too much.

14. Take Pictures of Yourself Throughout the Diet

I know you don't want to look, but think of this: Everyone else has to. Really. You're the only one who doesn't know how you look. You shouldn't be an ostrich with your head in the sand. Take the photos before you start your diet, and keep the picture in your head (or in your wallet) always. There is a bright side. After the first time, the pictures can only get better, and they'll help give you positive reinforcement to stay on the program.

15. Look in Mirrors
I'm not talking about the mirror in your compact. I'm talking about a full-length mirror.

My nearsighted friend Melvyn started running when he was in his mid-forties. He was heading back to his apartment the first week at about 7:30 A.M. when he saw a peculiar figure coming toward him. He was a little nervous, but didn't think the guy would hurt him. He looked pretty bad—his face was twisted, his hair was going in every direction, and he was dressed in old clothes. "He's probably a drug addict," Melvyn figured. When he was about three feet away, he realized he was looking in a mirror.

I scared myself, too. Shortly before I started the diet, I went to a party and had a couple of cocktails. That gave me the courage to come home and take off my clothes and stand in front of the mirror naked. Until that moment, I thought the most terrifying thing I'd ever seen was the shark scene in *Jaws*. I can joke about it now, but it was one of the things that convinced me to go on the diet. Now I like what I see; it's one of the things that helps keep me on the program.

16. Take Your Measurements
My overweight friend Judy was bragging about her little girl. "She has ribs," Judy said, "which haven't been seen in my family for generations." Ribs weren't the only part of my body that had gone into obscurity. I barely remembered something called "hollows" of the neck. Even in my mind's eye, I couldn't picture what my knees looked like in the aerial view.

You'll see the difference in your clothes, but if you're like me, you need as much reinforcement as possible. So before you begin, take a deep breath and take your measurements. Actually, you'd better let that deep breath out before you look at the tape measure.

So what if your thigh measures one and a half times Scarlett O'Hara's waist? Remember, this is the worst it's going to be. From now on, things will only get better.

Repeat the measurement as you go from step to step, or if you stay on one step for a while, measure every two weeks. You'll be surprised.

17. Weigh Only Once a Week

The most exercise I used to get was dragging the scale around the room trying to find a spot where I'd weigh the least. Who was I trying to kid? The only thing lower than fooling yourself about how much you weigh is cheating at solitaire.

Addicted dieters tend to go off the deep end if a day passes with no weight loss. "What the hell," they say to themselves, "nothing much is happening so I might as well eat this side of beef."

If you've made the commitment to the diet, you're in it for the long haul. You know your weight varies from day to day, so weigh yourself only once a week, same day, same time. And without any clothes, please; no trying to persuade yourself that your sandals weigh six pounds. If you're sticking to the program, you'll see a loss.

18. Weigh and Measure Your Food

If you're so crazy to get at the scales, buy one to keep in the kitchen and weigh your food on it. A diet scale or even a small postal scale will do. Also, measure your food: A heaping tablespoon contains almost twice as much—and twice as many calories—as a level one.

Weighing food is the best way to learn to judge portions by sight so you can keep track of what you're eating even when you're eating out. Here's one trick that might help: A four-ounce piece of meat is about the same size as a pack of playing cards. And to gauge a half-cup measure, make a fist: A half cup is about the distance from the top of your middle finger to the bottom of your pinkie.

But as a rule, don't guess—weigh. If you were so good at guessing weight by looking, how could you have convinced yourself you'd only gained a couple of pounds since the last time you were on a scale. . . .

19. Don't Put Yourself Down

None of those posters with pigs pasted on the refrigerator, please. None of the gadgets that say, "You fat slob" when you open the refrigerator door. I had one of those, and I got so depressed that I went out and bought a second refrigerator. A moving man I knew once said, "The body is just the console for the mind." Underneath all the excess baggage is *you*—the same person who'll be there once it's gone. Start respecting yourself now, to get in practice. Imagine how good you'll feel when you've Helped Yourself.

20. Don't Be Self-Conscious

So you're fat. That's not a crime against humanity. And you're probably a nicer person because of it. Seriously: Didn't most of the nicest people you know start out as goofy-looking kids? As soon as it occurs to you that your looks aren't your strong suit, if you have any brains at all you usually start developing some other drawing card. While the lookers were out on dates, the rest of us were home practicing humility—or the flute.

21. Don't Obsess

Two friends of mine with some time on their hands decided to actually make the recipe for Mock Apple Pie that's on the Ritz Cracker box. You use no apples—just thirty-six Ritz Crackers. At a critical moment in the preparation, one of them discovered they were one cracker short. "It won't work," my other friend said. "With thirty-five you make a Mock *Strawberry* Pie." People on diets often think like that. If they eat three ounces instead of four, or four instead of three, the magic formula won't work.

That's not true, of course. Ideally, you follow a program exactly. Don't keep throwing in an extra ounce here and there—it only takes sixteen to make a pound. But if you can't persuade a restaurant to serve you exactly four ounces of chicken, or you've misplaced your spoon measure and you have to guess at a half tablespoon of diet mayonnaise, the world won't come to an end, and neither will your diet.

22. Shop After You've Eaten

Or you'll go through that supermarket like Pac-Man. Supermarkets are in business to make money, and they're very good at it. They know how to get your mouth watering no matter how full you are. In the old days, I used to go out and buy some sweet rolls, bring them home, sprinkle cinnamon in a little tin pan, and burn it on the stove. Once you got a whiff, you thought I'd been baking all day. That's what they do in the supermarkets. I call it Faking Baking. Don't let them fool you. What you're smelling probably isn't being made on the premises. It was probably flown in from L.A., where they can't even give it away because all the people out there are so thin.

23. Shop with a List

You'll save calories and money, too. No impulse buying. And try and shop around the edges of the supermarket. That's where they usually have the fruits, the vegetables, the meats, the dairy products, and the bread. Once you're in the aisles, you're in trouble. That's where they keep the cookies and candy, the "convenience" food and junk. Plead fatigue and see if you can get the manager to bring you the cereal, then buy all your cleaning stuff and paper supplies at the discount drugstore.

24. Be Suspicious of Food That's Not Where It Should Be

Supermarkets know about merchandising. That's why you're walking along looking for your Diet Pepsi and you come upon the Doritos in a little display carton alongside it. Or you head for your strawberries and you find the cake shells and whipped cream, nowhere near where they should be. Supermarkets generally push snack foods—foods that aren't essential or important nutritionally—in this fashion. Notice they don't do it with foods generally regarded as good for you. I've never seen anyone display onions together with the liver.

25. Start Reading the Labels on Food

You look inside your dresses, don't you? You sneak a look under your hostess's plate to see what brand of china she's using. Why aren't you looking to find out what's going into your mouth?

I bought a frozen dessert from a strolling vendor because he told me it was made with skim milk and real fruit. Low-cal, I thought. As I peeled off the wrapper, I noticed that among the ingredients were heavy cream and corn syrup. And the vendor had such an honest-looking face. . . .

Lay off the canned and processed food: It's full of salt and sugar and additives, as you'll know once you read the labels.

You'll come across some other eye-openers. For example, you should know that the ingredients are listed in order: whatever there's most of comes first, whatever there's next most of is second, and so forth. A lot of cleaning products list "aqueous solution" as the first ingredient. "Aqueous solution" is just water. Water is also the primary ingredient in a lot of "fruit" drinks. I wonder how many people realize that "all-natural" fruit drinks are often 10 percent fruit, plus water and fructose—it may be natural, because it's not made in a laboratory, but it's sugar.

You should lay off the juices anyway. One eight-ounce glass is the equivalent of two or more pieces of the real thing. If Nature meant you to get fruit two or three pieces at a time, the serpent would have offered Eve a can and a straw.

26. When You Get the Eating Out of the Closet, Take Your Fat Clothes Along with It

Get rid of those fat clothes. They're just a setup for failure. You figure if the diet doesn't work out, your roomy clothes will take you back in. They're your enemy. Give them away. Donate them to the Salvation Army. If you have a lot of weight to lose, I know it's going to be difficult to manage a wardrobe. But you can certainly alter your larger things. Not only will they look better, but you'll be encouraged to keep going. Once a tailor takes out a couple of inches of a dart, there's no going back. Also, buy just a few inexpensive things in your new size—maybe a pair of pants and two or three blouses. You need and deserve to feel good. At the very least, you can always get a belt for the dresses you just used to let hang. You'll be happy about every new notch.

27. Wear Form-fitting Clothes

My idea of a person who looks good in a tent is Lawrence of Arabia. I've been there. Not to Arabia, but in a lot of those tent dresses. I had enough tent dresses to hold a good-sized lawn party underneath them. Now here's the sad truth. Those dresses just make you look heavier. Get out of your "float." (I love that euphemism. The dress designers must have had a good laugh choosing it. As everyone knows, a float is a large moving object that belongs in a parade.) Just because you're not wearing a belt, you're not fooling anyone. The opposite may be true: Those dresses are an obvious attempt to hide fat.

Start wearing clothes that reveal your body. For one thing, when you try and fit into clothes with zippers and waistlines, you're forced to take a good look at yourself and honestly figure out how much you should lose. In the second place, as your fat starts to disappear, your friends will notice sooner. You deserve to be complimented.

28. Get a Proxy Eater

Society women often show up on the arms of "walkers" who escort them to parties while their husbands are busy making the bucks.

While I recommend you exercise alone, I can see the benefit of a walker to take to parties. While you're at it, get an eater, too. That's a person who comes along with you and eats all the stuff you'd like to but can't. I always get a vicarious thrill from a proxy eater, who is ideally a very thin person with a high metabolic rate.

My friend Joanie is an executive who has to go on a lot of expense account lunches, and she found that some people were uncomfortable when she was dieting and eating 400-calorie lunches, and they were not. She started bringing her assistant Heather along as a proxy eater so her guests wouldn't have to indulge alone. Joanie lost her weight, but Heather, who hadn't been eating expense account lunches till then, ate so much rich food that she worked herself out of her size 8's and up to size 18's. She moved to Hawaii, where she's known as Honolulu Heather, the Muumuu Mama. I'm sending her a copy of the Help Yourself program.

29. In Restaurants, Don't Read the Menu

It's not as if you're an extraterrestial. You know your way around a menu. You've been in a restaurant before. You pretty much know what the place is going to have. Make up your mind what you should be eating without looking at the menu—broiled fish, steak, baked chicken, green salad with no dressing, vegetables. Sure there will come a time when you can eat like a thin person, but while you're trying to stay within a caloric limit, you're better off keeping it simple. I'd stay out of ethnic restaurants in the beginning of a diet if I were in your situation—which I have been, of course.

30. Don't Take Any Guff from Waiters

Most waiters and waitresses are pretty good eggs, but every once in a while you run into one of those characters straight out of *Five Easy Pieces* who told Jack Nicholson he couldn't get toast. (Remember what he did? He ordered chicken salad. On white bread. *Toasted* white bread. Then, as the waitress headed for the kitchen, he added, "And hold the chicken salad.")

Don't let yourself be intimidated in restaurants. Just keep telling yourself that in most restaurants, particularly if they have a bar, they've seen everything. Now, I'm not advising, as they do on a certain other diet that's floating around, that you hand the waiter or waitress a little piece of paper with a list of foods you would like, most of which probably aren't on the menu. That's just asking for a smart remark.

131

On the other hand, asking to substitute a vegetable for the potato or requesting that your fish be broiled without butter shouldn't get a rude response. I remind you of this because I know that fat people are often shy about asserting themselves in restaurants. They secretly feel everyone is thinking, What are you doing here anyway? You've had enough to eat in your life already.

31. A1 Sauce Is the Dieter's Best Friend
Not on steak. On layer cake. If you're tempted to nibble when you've had enough, or when there's something on the plate that you absolutely should not eat, put A1 sauce over it. Of course I understand that for lunch President Ford topped his cottage cheese with A1 because he actually preferred it that way, but for me, putting A1 sauce on anything but meat is the kiss of death. Alternative: Pour on the salt. It may not be the suavest move you'll ever make in a restaurant, but who cares?

32. Start Learning About Nutrition
Even though I'd like to, I can't cram everything you should know about the subject between the covers of this book. There are libraries full of information. You might want to start with Jane Brody's *Nutrition Book*, which is one of the best books around. As a side benefit, you're better off reading Jane Brody than one of those gothic romances. You'll be improving your mind along with your body, and you'll have something to talk about at cocktail parties instead of circling around the buffet. Just be careful that with all your newfound information you don't make the hostess feel too guilty about serving all the liquor and the hors d'oeuvres spiked with MSG that cause brain damage.

33. Don't Serve Meals in Serving Platters
Serve yourself and your family in the kitchen—or near the stove if you eat in the kitchen—giving everyone the appropriate amount. Avoid the temptation of having a heaping bowlful of anything right in front of your dinner plate. If your family wants seconds, let them go back into the kitchen for them. The walk will probably do them good.

34. Discuss Food or Dieting Only While You're Eating
Did you ever notice that slim people unselfconsciously discuss what

they're eating, while fat people discuss what they're not eating? ("I only had six ounces of cottage cheese all day." Of course, sometimes they lie.) Both subjects are relatively boring once you've left the dining room and therefore should not be discussed unless you're a member of a culinary society, which I would definitely not advise. Take up another hobby, like skin-diving. It's hard to snack under water.

35. When It's Over, It's Over

"Tomorrow" should be your new theme song. There's always tomorrow to start eating some more. When you've finished a meal, put your fork down and get away from the table—fast. Clear the dishes off, and get out of the room. Preferably you'll get right out of the house and take a moderate walk.

36. Don't Hang Around the Kitchen

Get out of there. If you're in the kitchen, I'd bet it's not to admire the wallpaper. Allow yourself a run-through only. The less time you spend surrounded by food and food accessories, the better. This goes not only for your kitchen, but other people's. Sit in the garden; sit in the living room. Don't even offer to help clean up at parties. Let other people do it for a change.

37. Rehearse High-Risk Situations

When I was anticipating a special occasion, I used to think beforehand about what I was going to eat. I still do, only now it takes me a lot less time because there's a lot less I plan to eat. I actually try and picture myself in a situation that I know will be difficult—a party, a holiday dinner, a meal in a favorite restaurant—and I decide very specifically what I will do. If I've decided I'll have two drinks, I follow a plan and drink them on schedule. Otherwise, I might conveniently "forget" how many I've had and go overboard. It's also very easy to overeat when friends urge you to join them, unless you've decided ahead of time that you will stay in control and made up your mind how.

38. Keep Those Emergency Stores Out of the House

I once calculated that if three dozen refugees landed on my doorstep in the middle of the night, I could serve them four brownies apiece. If they didn't land, I had plenty of brownies for myself. I didn't even have to go through the trouble of baking them. I could just eat the mix right from the package or dust my vanilla ice cream with it.

I had a friend who really loved birthday cake. He'd go around town ordering cakes—"Happy Birthday, Barry," "Happy Birthday, Brad," and so forth—then go home and eat them by himself. He started freezing the cakes, so he wouldn't eat them all at once. Then he discovered that the best place for food to thaw is in your stomach.

Anything fattening that's lying around the house, I discovered, soon wound up in my mouth. While you still haven't gotten control of your eating, keep it out. I read some diet tips about storing the fattening food out of sight, in the back of the cabinet. What I want to know is what it's doing there in the first place. If you're worried about your friends coming over and finding the cupboard bare, maybe this is a good time to think about who your friends are, anyway. Are they coming for your companionship . . . or your cake? More important: Are you keeping the stuff for them . . . or for yourself?

39. When the Guests Leave, the Party's Over

I think a really pathetic sight is a guy wearing a party hat standing in an empty room, in the middle of a pile of dirty plates, stuffing his face with cold cuts. Once your friends have gone home, throw away everything that hasn't been eaten. If you can't bear to do that, wrap up the food and send it home with your guests as if it were wedding cake. Tell them they'll be doing you a big favor by getting it out of the house. Otherwise, the leftover will turn into a hangover—the kind that hangs over your belt.

40. Find a New Hangout

As a rule of thumb, stay away from any place where the waitress says to you, "Can I bring you the usual?" If I know you, the usual is not a watercress sandwich. Certain places trigger certain kinds of behavior. If your hangout is the local pub, you're going to be awfully tempted to order your favorite cocktail; or maybe your weakness is the apple pie at the diner. Stay away until you're really in control.

41. Don't Join a Fancy Health Club

As if it isn't discouraging enough to have to sign those releases absolving blame if the program sends you out the door feet first, you also have to cope with the instructors. Those same people who chose you last for their teams in high school are now supposed to be helping you get into shape, and it's been my experience they're about as sympathetic and helpful as Miss Hannigan was to Little Orphan Annie. I have always felt that fancy health clubs are really just places where people obsessed with their bodies can show them off when it isn't nice enough to go to the beach. There are exceptions, of course, but as a rule, if you want to add another kind of exercise to your walking, I think you're better off joining your local Y. Many of them have excellent programs with realistic expectations, and they're not expensive.

42. Avoid Diet Schemes

If somebody you meet at a party tried to get you to back the Gordon Liddy Tranquility Institute, you'd think he was crazy. Then how come when Cousin Suzie from Hoboken shows up at Thanksgiving with another of her loony diets you turn into a turkey, too? You start taking notes about some wild program that involves watermelon and horseradish and you're ready to start following it like the Holy Grail.

You know that song "My Way"? I think it should be the theme song for dieters. Everybody's got another method that's going to get those twenty pounds off you fast and forever. One thing I can assure you: If it happens fast, it won't be forever.

Do yourself a favor. You've already spent the money on this book. Follow the program. It's going to work. Then when you see Counsin Suzie next Thanksgiving, if she hasn't already gone to her Great Reward in the Sky from the botulism in her diet protein shake, you can lend her this book so she can start losing the weight she's gained since last year.

43. Remember That a Diet Is Not a Punishment

It's not great having to write down all your calories and keep exercising. But consider the alternatives. Do you enjoy living in bed and having your view of your toes blocked by your stomach? Lying down is a good place to examine how overweight you truly are, since in that position your fat is generally distributed as evenly as possible. I knew I was in trouble when I couldn't locate my hipbones when I was flat on my back. Don't be mad that you're on a diet. Remember you had a pretty good time before you started. Now try telling yourself that a diet is not something you're *enduring*, it's something you're *doing*. Be proud of yourself and think how great it will be to live like a lean and fit person.

44. Don't Believe Your Mother

That very same woman who told you that there was a Santa Claus, that the stork brought babies, and that you were prettier than any Miss America is now telling you that you look too thin. Don't believe her. Unfortunately, well-meaning moms, along with loving friends and devoted spouses, have a hard time accepting a fitter you when they're used to a fatter you. Give them some time to get used to the new way you look. It is possible to diet to excess, but if you follow the Help Yourself program—particularly the part about adding calories—you will be eating properly and you will be at a weight that is appropriate and healthy for you.

Part Three

Second Helpings

Second Helpings are for people who haven't had enough. I'm hoping that includes you. It includes me: At this point in the book I still haven't had a chance to share all the things I've discovered about food, nutrition, and exercise. That's why I've added this section.

Some of the questions in Q&A are ones I myself asked Dr. Joel. Fiction/Fact includes some of my favorite (wrong) notions that I've now been corrected on. Did You Know That? . . . is full of facts you should know, and Other Ways to Fry a Fish, which is not about frying fish, is full of cooking suggestions I think you'll find useful. And that's just a part of what Second Helpings is about.

Nibbles comes first, because for dieters, nibbles have to go first! I know it seems hard: When I first swore off pecan sandies, I wondered what would get me out of bed in the morning! I don't get my kicks from cookies anymore. I get them from feeling great about myself.

Chapter 14

Nibbles

Do you think about food too much? Try this word association test and find out.

Tonsillectomy	a) Operation	b) Ice cream
Picnic	a) Ants	b) Potato salad
Weddings	a) Brides	b) Cake
Ronald Reagan	a) Washington	b) Jelly beans
Romance	a) Valentines	b) Chocolates
Circus	a) Clown	b) Cotton candy
Virility	a) Warren Beatty	b) Oysters
Mom	a) Pop	b) Apple pie
Pop	a) Mom	b) Soda
Illness	a) Doctors	b) Chicken soup

*   *   *

The World's Most Fattening Beverage: Eggnog has 335 calories per four-ounce serving.

*   *   *

The Pilgrims got their first taste of popcorn at the first Thanksgiving dinner—which, by the way, was really a breakfast served by chief Massasoit's brother to the Pilgrims and ninety-two members of his tribe. Dessert was popcorn, which I believe everyone ate plain. So should you. Here's why:

Popcorn, one cup dry: 40 calories
Popcorn, one cup popped with fat and salt: 81 calories
Popcorn, one cup popped with a sugar coating: 134 calories.

*   *   *

At one-half teaspoon per stick, 60 percent of a stick of gum is pure sugar. Nineteen percent is cornstarch. One stick of gum has about 9 calories. Sugarless gum has about 8 calories per stick.

A few brands of sugarless gum are sweetened with "aspartame"—a sweetener that's about twenty-one times as potent as sugar. Four calories worth of aspartame, though, is as sweet as two teaspoons of sugar (36 calories). So far, it hasn't been okayed for use in sodas, but it will appear in cold breakfast cereals, puddings, dessert toppings, and other products.

* * *

Flavor of the month: Pickled Plum chewing gum, a Japanese chaw.

* * *

The party's over . . . before the main course, if you hit the hors d'oeuvres tables. A strolling snacker can take in as many calories as if she's eaten a full-course meal. Check the chart below before you run for the cocktail plate:

Item	Calories
3 Triscuits	63
with	
1 ounce-cheddar cheese (enough for 3 crackers)	112
2 chicken livers wrapped in bacon	180
1 fried chicken wing	54
2 Vienna link frankfurters	78
3 Wheat Thins	27
with	
1 ounce chicken liver pâté	80
10 peanuts	105
	689

* * *

It may be a once-a-year thing, but the party's still over . . . if you nibble on these "occasional" foods. Maybe it's a birthday, a company bash, an engagement party. The merrymaker may make herself miserable the next day just remembering how she celebrated a happy event. Check the figures below before you lift a forkful:

Item	Calories
8 ounces champagne	164
1 ounce Brie cheese	94
with	

140

Item *(cont'd.)*	Calories
3 sesame crackers	45
1 ounce Cheese Puffs	158
3 spareribs with barbecue sauce	168
1 serving of vanilla ice cream	145
with	
1 piece of yellow cake with chocolate icing	163
	937

* * *

Blame the Swiss: Milk chocolate was first made in Switzerland in 1876.

* * *

The Reverend Sylvester W. Graham (for whom the cracker was named) was a onetime preacher and food faddist who believed that pepper, mustard, and ketchup caused insanity.

I wouldn't go that far. Pepper's a respectable spice. In fact, hot red pepper has more vitamin C per ounce than any other fruit or vegetable. (Only the Human Torch could knock back an ounce of the fiery stuff.) Although a sprinkling of black pepper doesn't boast a high vitamin content, it does add snap to foods, with barely any calories. Mustard is actually a blend of mustard seed or powder, flour, and other spices in a base of either water, wine, vinegar, or champagne. Mustard has about 4 calories per teaspoon. Ketchup averages about 20 calories per tablespoon, depending on the brand, not because of the main ingredient (tomatoes), but because of the sugar content. Some ketchups are about one-third to one-quarter sugar.

* * *

America's favorite side order is french fried potatoes. Ten fries, about 2″ × ½″ × ½″, have 156 calories. Who eats just ten?

* * *

Ga-ga over goobers: The average person consumes about 3½ pounds of peanut butter a year. In fact, I suspect that most people eat none, while all the rest is consumed by kids and the moms who make their sandwiches. Three tablespoons of peanut butter have 288 calories and 23.9 grams of fat.

Peanuts are nutritious, but fattening. Three-quarters of an ounce of salted peanuts gives you 105 calories and 10.7 grams of fat—about a quarter of a day's allowance. Sugar plus nuts are a caloric double whammy: Peanut brittle has 128 calories per 1-ounce piece. Don't go nuts with nuts.

* * *

You have 9000 taste buds on your tongue. Nature was very clever in placing them: the tip determines sweetness, the sides, salt. The taste buds for picking up sourness are located farther back on the sides; bitterness is picked up way back on your tongue. These are the four basic tastes with shades between them.

Before it's on the tip of your tongue, reconsider your breakfast order: Do you really want that jelly doughnut (226 calories)?

* * *

I hate to admit this, but . . . pizza is not just "empty calories." It's a pretty nutritious nibble. Experts say it's fairly well-balanced for fast food, with protein, carbohydrates, fat, vitamin A, and some minerals. Still, one 217-calorie slice is about 27 percent fat.

The thicker the crust and the more pepperoni and/or anchovies are laid on, the more the calories and fat content go up. Pizza is an okay *snack* for a growing teenager to eat. Pizza, for you and me, is a *meal*.

* * *

Speaking of fast food: I didn't grow up with Whoppers or Dairy Queen Cheese Dogs and you probably didn't either. Burger and malt shops, pizza parlors and ice-cream joints were around then, but not lying in wait on every corner the way they are today.

Fast food places are great once in a while, more as a matter of convenience than as "restaurants" that serve balanced meals. The food you get in fast food shops is high in protein, but also high in fat and salt—and if you go for the straw-clogging thick malts, high in sugar, too.

Fast food menus are low (or lacking) in fresh fruit dishes and cooked vegetables. Don't expect to find low-cal nibbles. Even a dish that sounds as if it might be for a dieter, like Poppin' Fresh's Chef's Salad, has 800 calories, 40 more than a Whopper with cheese.

* * *

Fourteen reasons to nibble and/or binge you should never use again:

You're worried
It's that time of month
You're lonely
You just had a fight
You can always diet
You're frustrated
You're bored
You're nervous

You don't want to waste food others have left over
You're going through a crisis
It's "health" food so it's good for you
You need a pep up
You're happy
It's there

* * *

Dubious designer binge: When asked by *Cosmopolitan*, "What do you do when you go on a binge?" Gloria Vanderbilt replied: "Cinnamon on cottage cheese. I pretend it's rice pudding."

* * *

The fourth biggest lie: One size fits all.

Chapter 15

Q&A

What's the difference between low-cal and reduced calorie foods? How can you tell which fish is fattiest before biting into it? Answers to these questions and others you've wondered about follow. . . .

Q: Help! I loved the diets that let you eat all the meat you wanted. Now you tell me to eat only five ounces of steak. That isn't much.

A: An eight-ounce T-bone steak, broiled, has 545 calories. Not great. Worse yet, it seems that a diet high in fat and protein may pose a greater risk of cancer than cigarette smoking. The word comes from a Cornell University nutritionist.

The typical American gets 40–50 percent of his calories from fats. Ideally, a government Committee on Nutrition and Human Needs has found, the typical American should get 50–65 percent from carbohydrates, 15–20 percent from protein, and 20–30 percent from fats. Studies show that fat intake exceeding 35 percent of total calories is associated with cancers of the colon, prostate, breast, and large bowel. Diet may be the most important risk factor for cancer.

The diet recommended to decrease the risk of cancer is the same one that has been associated with a decreased likelihood of cardiovascular disease and diabetes.

This should discourage you from making meat the mainstay of your diet—whether or not you're trying to cut calories. You're eating meat out of habit, and you need to reeducate yourself to control the food. The food shouldn't control you.

Q: Okay. Now that I know about limiting my intake of beef, won't I be spending more to buy the cheaper cuts? Don't they have less fat than the cheaper ones?

A: Not at all. Beef is graded by fat content and the results are just the opposite of what you think. The better the cut of meat, the *higher* the fat content. Here's how the grading breaks down: *prime:*

40–50 percent of total weight is fat; *choice:* 35–40 percent of total weight is fat; *good:* 25–35 of total weight is fat.

Hamburger, by law, must be 30–35 percent fat. A lot of fat melts out when you cook hamburger. Broil it so fat drips off into the pan below.

Lean ground beef, generally ground from chuck or rump, is about 20–25 percent fat.

Extra lean beef, about 15–20 percent fat, is your best buy. You lose less volume because of fat melting out and end up with more lean beef.

If you're preparing beef for the family, choose chuck, rump, or round. They are generally lower in saturated fats than prime ribs, sirloin, and porterhouse.

Q: Is all fish low in calories?

A: Fish is not only categorized by whether it's fresh or saltwater bred, but also (among other qualities) by size, shape, and fat content. Generally, you can spot the fattier fish in a flash—the darker the flesh, the higher the fat content.

A fattier-fleshed fish is better suited to grilling or roasting because of the extra oil in it. A leaner-fleshed fish is generally cooked in oil or butter—which may bring the calorie count up to more than a same-sized serving of a fattier cousin. Instead, broil or steam it.

Here are a few examples of fatty vs. less fatty fish per 3½-ounce serving, uncooked, based on statistics from the United States Department of Agriculture:

Atlantic salmon: 217 calories
Rainbow trout: 195 calories
Shad: 170 calories
Pacific mackerel: 159 calories
Bluefin tuna: 145 calories
Weakfish: 121 calories
Bluefish: 117 calories
Striped bass: 105 calories
Whiting: 105 calories
Atlantic and Pacific halibut: 100 calories
Sturgeon: 94 calories
Red snapper: 93 calories
Yellow perch: 91 calories
Tilefish: 79 calories
Cod: 78 calories

Here's a piece of information to drop at dinner parties: The tail end of the fish has a more intense flavor because of the exercise the fish gets from swimming around, but the tail meat's a bit less tender than the rest.

Q: I've seen tofu at the market. What is it?

A: Tofu is a low-calorie, fairly nutritious soybean cake that's a good, inexpensive vegetable protein source. Tofu is made by mashing soybeans into soymilk, then pressing the curd mixture into a solid cake. Tofu has about 9.4 grams of protein in a two-inch square, no cholesterol, minimal saturated fat, and 72 calories for 3½ ounces.

Once these soybean cakes were only available in Oriental markets. Now they can be found, usually next to the bean sprouts, in the produce section of your supermarket. For about 30–35¢ a cake, you get a bargain in nutrition.

Q: What's the difference between "reduced calorie" food and "low calorie" foods?

A: When a food is labeled "reduced calories," there must be one-third fewer calories per serving than a comparable food made by another company. If a food is labeled "low calorie," you should be getting no more than 40 calories per serving—that's the law.

Q: Aren't pasta, potatoes, and bread no-nos on a diet?

A: You've been scared off from all carbohydrates—wrongly. Carbohydrates come in two forms. One is simple sugars, which are absorbed right into your system with a minimal amount of processing to give you instant energy. When instant energy supplies run out, you still need energy.

You get it from the other form of carbohydrates: starches. They are just complex sugars that take longer to process than simple sugars. The breakdown of starch helps keep you from feeling fatigued. If your body is short of carbohydrates, it will begin to break down muscle (protein) to make simple sugars. *This* is a no-no.

Q: Aren't condensed milk and evaporated milk the same?

A: No more than malted milk and skim milk! A tablespoon of condensed milk has 64 calories, thanks to the added sugar. Evaporated has 22, whole milk (3.25 percent fat) has 11, and skim has 5 per tablespoon. Some people think evaporated skim milk tastes "richer" in coffee than skim and gives the coffee a better color. Try it.

Q: Can I eat sugarless mints and gum?

A: You're suppose to break the habit of eating—or having something in your mouth—between meals. Besides, some folks suffer gas attacks from "sugarless" mints or gum that contains xylitol or sorbitol. If you blame that slightly bloated feeling on whatever you ate before you popped a mint, think again.

Cause of the gas? We can't digest certain carbohydrates. When they hit the intestines, bacteria that live there ferment the undigested stuff and, bingo—gas. Beans have the dubious honor of creating the most of this stuff. Other culprits: cabbage, spinach, grapes, cereal bran, and even innocent-seeming apple juice.

Q: If I exercise an hour every day, do I have to cut calories, too?
A: Farah Fawcett once said that since she exercises so much, she eats all she wants. If you follow the plan, some day you too will be able to eat like Farah, though I can't guarantee you'll *look* like her. If you're just starting the program, let me remind you that exercising without cutting caloric intake *will* eventually lead to a weight loss. The key word is *eventually*. No dieter I know was ever interested in *slow* weight loss. So cut your calories while you exercise and you'll get to your goal that much quicker.

Q: How long do I need to exercise before I know I'm burning body fat, not just losing water by perspiring?
A: Obviously, when you exercise strenuously you begin to perspire. The reason you sweat during exercise is the same reason you sweat when the weather's hot—it's your body's way of cooling you down. After about fifteen minutes of exercise, if you really work at it, you begin to perspire. After half an hour to forty-five minutes, you are using body fat for energy and fuel.

In case you wondered: The average woman's brain weighs forty-four ounces; the average man's, forty-nine ounces. When you're not exercising, your brain uses 66 percent of the glucose in your body, while your muscles divide up the rest. Your less-than-three-pound brain uses up as much glucose as some thirty-to-seventy pounds of muscle (depending on your body size).

Chapter 16

Fact/Fiction

There's an old superstition that thunderstorms curdle milk. This is only true if the storm causes power failure and your refrigerator, with milk in it, shuts off. Other myths about food (and your body) need some clearing up, too.

Fiction: Grapefruit and pineapple will burn body fat.

Fact: Over the years, grapefruit has been the main ingredient in several "miracle" reducing plans. It's a fine food, with few calories and plenty of vitamin C, but it doesn't burn body fat. Same for pineapple. No such fat-burning food has yet been discovered. When it is, I'm buying it all.

Fiction: Converted rice and enriched rice have the same nutritional value, while wild rice has more calories.

Fact: Converted rice is parboiled and heat-treated before it is dried, milled, and packaged. Heat treating draws the nutrients from the rice bran and germ into the grain. When white rice is processed, the bran and germ are removed. White rice then may be "enriched" with some nutrients (after being stripped of them), but it's not as nutritious as converted rice. It's also higher in calories.

Wild rice has fewer calories per serving than either white or brown rice. A quarter cup of raw, wild rice has 99 calories. Brown rice has 176 calories, white enriched has 178 calories, and converted has 114 calories. Wild rice also has more protein, magnesium, and phosphorus. Unfortunately, wild rice is much more expensive than the others.

Fiction: Bananas are fattening.

Fact: Compared to apples and oranges, the banana is sweeter: a ripe banana is about 21 percent sugar, an apple 14 percent sugar, and an orange 12 percent. Yet the average 3½-ounce (6″) banana has only 85 calories. A medium apple has 80 calories and an orange has 80 calories.

That 3½-ounce banana has 1.1 grams of protein and plenty of potassium, but no cholesterol—good for healthy hearts. Bananas also have a very mild laxative effect—the fiber and pectin in the fruit purportedly aid in curbing constipation. It takes your system three hours to digest a banana.

In case you wondered if there were any banana-holics around, the answer's yes. Natives of Buganda, Uganda, are bananas over bananas. According to *The Total Banana* by Alex Abella, the average Bugandan consumes about 9 (nine) pounds (pounds) of bananas per day—that's about 2½ bananas per waking hour.

Fiction: "Sugar-free" foods are less caloric than those with sugar.

Fact: No such luck. "Sugar free" only means that there's no sugar in the product—the manufacturer wasn't pulling your leg on that. However, it doesn't mean that what you're buying isn't loaded with other sweeteners which are *as* caloric or *more* caloric than sugar. Ice creams or desserts flavored with honey may have more calories because honey has more calories per teaspoon than sugar. Corn sweeteners, corn syrup, fructose, sorbitol, and molasses are other high caloric additions. When you buy something that says it's sugar free, compare the calorie count to a similar product made with sugar. Of course, the sweetest reward comes from being able to pass the stuff by, sugar free or not.

Fiction: There are fewer calories in a pound of whipped butter or margarine than in the nonwhipped stick or tub varieties.

Fact: There are fewer calories in the whipped stuff *only if you use less of it*. One pound of whipped margarine has the same calorie count as a pound of nonwhipped margarine.

When margarine is whipped, you get a larger *volume* per pound since whipping adds air. The trick is to use less. The smaller the serving, the fewer the calories.

Fiction: Margarine has fewer calories than butter.

Fact: By law, butter must have a fat content of 80 percent. The same law applies to margarine—it's 80 percent fat. Margarine usually has no cholesterol since it's not made with saturated fats (like lard) but with vegetable oils.

Here's the catch. Unsaturated vegetable oils become somewhat saturated when they've been hydrogenated or partially hydrogenated, the process that makes them solid. You wind up with 100 calories per tablespoon for both butter or margarine. Whipped margarine has about 65 calories per tablespoon.

Diet margarines have less fat and more water content, therefore, lower calories. Diet margarines are about 40 percent fat and 55 calories per tablespoon.

Fiction: Foods like celery and apples have "negative calories" because of the energy needed to chew and digest them.

Fact: A calorie is a calorie is a calorie, whether you're eating apples or strawberry shortcake. An average-size person uses only 0.3 calories per minute while eating. That means a 5-calorie stalk of celery would have to be chewed for seventeen minutes to have no caloric value. I imagine you have better things to do.

Fiction: Eggplant is a meat substitute.

Fact: Only by reputation. Like most vegetables, eggplant is mostly water. In fact, it's 93 percent water. Four percent of this vegetable is carbohydrate.

Eggplant is probably thought of as a meat substitute because it's commonly used in a popular dish, eggplant Parmigiana. This vegetable has certain physical qualities that make it practical to use in such a recipe. It can be sliced into "steaks," breaded, and fried without falling apart—under a watchful eye. Eggplant also works like a blotter—it soaks up cooking oil as it loses its water content when in the pan.

A half cup of eggplant, cooked with no oil, has only 38 calories and about 2 grams of protein. Add bread crumbs, cheese, and fry in oil, and the calorie count and fat content soar. Don't blame it on the eggplant.

Fiction: Your stomach shrinks as you diet.

Fact: When you diet successfully, you become accustomed to eating less food. Your stomach is the same size as always.

Fiction: Using "nondairy" creamers or dessert toppings save calories.

Fact: Sorry. Nondairy creamers have more calories per tablespoon than milk since most of them are made with coconut oil. Coconut has the highest saturated fat content per gram of any other vegetable oil. Coffee-mate has 21.7 percent saturated fats and 11 calories per teaspoon.

Many dessert toppings are made from coconut oil, too. Richwhip and Cool Whip are high in saturated fats. Richwhip has 20 calories per tablespoon and Cool Whip 19.

Fiction: Lecithin pills burn fat.

Fact: Sorry, not a chance. Lecithin is a fat. Your body reacts to commercially made lecithin pills as it would to other fats: It breaks it down and sends it through your system. Here's the surprise: Lecithin pills have calories—in fact, 9 calories per pill.

Chapter 17

Did You Know That? . . .

Thomas Jefferson, our third President, was responsible for importing to America rice, the waffle iron, Calcutta hogs, Neapolitan macaroni, French wines, french fries, ice cream, mustard, Parmesan cheese, vanilla, olive oil, asparagus, and broccoli. Other facts about food, fat, and exercise may be just as surprising to you. For example, did you know that:

• White meat roasted turkey and dark meat roasted chicken have the same calorie count (176 calories per 3½ ounces), but dark meat turkey is about 40 percent fattier.

* * *

• Canadian bacon is lower in calories and fat content than the cured American variety, but is about 30–40 percent saltier.

* * *

• Artichokes, rich in potassium and iron, have only 44 calories per cooked globe (base and soft ends of the leaves). If you just like the hearts, skip the ones swimming in jars of oil, and head for the frozen food section. Frozen artichoke hearts, without oil, have only 26 calories per 3½ ounces! Add a few to a salad. Another plus: One artichoke contains 4 times the fiber of a bran muffin.

* * *

• Water-packed tuna has about 20 percent more protein and up to 161 fewer calories per 3½-ounce serving than oil-packed. Water-packed tuna is about 99 percent protein and 1 percent fat. Tuna gives you three to four times the niacin (which helps break down starch and sugar, so important in dieting) and one-fourth more vitamin B_{12} (which helps your blood cells carry oxygen, important in exercising) than steak.

* * *

• Cooking sherry of the supermarket variety contains about one teaspoon of salt per cup, plus other flavorings and additives. By law, cooking sherry should not appeal to consumers as an alcoholic beverage—it must be undrinkable as is. (I have some distant cousins who could ignore this feature.) Calories per cup: 76.

* * *

• Dry roasted peanuts have just about the same amount of calories as cocktail peanuts cooked in oil. A lot.

* * *

• If you use plain low-fat yogurt instead of sour cream, you save about 273 calories per cup.

* * *

• Lean rump roast has fewer calories and a lower fat count than lean roasted leg of lamb. Two slices of lamb: 107 calories and 3.5 grams of fat. Two slices of rump roast: 78 calories and 1.1 grams of fat.

* * *

• You may think you're saving tons of calories by eating sherbet instead of ice cream; you're not. You do get less fat with sherbet but you'll also be getting more sugar. One-half cup of sherbet equals 120–150 calories, depending on the flavor and the brand.

* * *

• At 61 calories a tablespoon, honey has more calories than sugar (46 calories a tablespoon).

* * *

• Except for unsalted or low-salt cottage cheese or any cheese made especially low in salt, *all* cheeses are high in sodium. How did the salt get in? Not only are salt and other sodium compounds added for flavor, they're also used to control acidity and curb undesirable bacterial growth. Some pasteurized processed cheeses are very high in sodium—up to 490 milligrams per ounce. (See Chapter 18, The Most Dangerous Things to Put in Your Mouth, for more on salt.)

*   *   *

• Vegetables that are steamed are more nutritious than vegetables cooked in water. It takes longer, though: Steam doesn't conduct heat as well as boiling water. As usual, patience is a virtue: You'll get more out of steamed vegetables.

*   *   *

• There's about 6 percent more sugar in frozen yogurt than in ice cream.

*   *   *

• Brie cheese imported to the United States has about a 50 percent fat content. Supposedly, Brie sold in France has only a 40 percent fat content. This is not a Gallic plot: It's just that pasteurized milk is used in the exported product.

*   *   *

• Broth, bouillon, and consommé are not the same thing, though they have identical calorie counts. Broth is the liquid that meat, vegetables, or grains have been cooked in. Broth is also called stock. Bouillon is a clear soup that's usually lightly seasoned. Consommé is often made from one or two kinds of meat. It too is a clear soup, but is highly seasoned. Beef broth, bouillon, or consommé have 23 calories per cup; chicken, 22 calories per cup. Go easy on commercially made soups like these: They tend to be on the salty side.

*   *   *

• Milk and other dairy products aren't the only good sources of calcium. Cabbage, broccoli, and kale are also rich sources. Calcium is especially important to women beginning in middle age, when they're candidates for the bone disorder osteoporosis.

* * *

• Pistachio nuts have 88 calories per 30 nuts. Cashews come in at 280 calories for between 20–26 nuts.

* * *

• When you see the words "nonnutritive crude fiber" listed in your cereal's ingredients, you're paying extra for, yes, *wood* fiber. Crude fiber won't make you sick, but neither do you need it. Fiber from grain and fruits, though, are another story. An increase in fiber is recommended by many doctors—fiber has been shown to regulate bowels and may decrease the risk of colon cancer.

* * *

• Seven Triscuits (at 21 calories each) have the same calorie count as a scoop of chocolate ice cream (147 calories).

* * *

• Though you might have been taught that vegetables that are yellow or reddish are high in vitamin A, it's not so with beets and radishes. One large carrot has 650 times as much vitamin A as two raw medium-sized beets and 11,000 times the vitamin A in ten radishes. Beets are also low in protein, vitamin C, and iron. For 43 calories (two beets), you get mostly flavor and a great color. However . . . beet greens are great. One cup is high in vitamin A, a good source of calcium, and provides one-third of your RDA of iron. Radishes are pretty low in nutrients—they have only that snappy taste and low calorie count going for them. Ten have 17 calories.

* * *

• Smaller Cornish hens, turkeys, and chickens are leaner than the larger ones.

* * *

• Depending on the type of mix you use (homemade or commercial), just under two-thirds or so of the calories (260–290) in an average slice of pie come from the top and bottom crusts alone. And you know why. The crust is flour, water, and fat—and of course, some sugar.

*   *   *

• Most sugar-free mints have about 8 calories each. Regular Tic-Tacs have 1½ calories each. If you'd buy sugar-free mints, such as Velamints, in bulk like candy, you'd pay about $6.50 a pound.

*   *   *

• Two highballs, Manhattans, or 12-ounce cans of beer (like Michelob) amount to 320 calories. That's nearly *one-third* of a dieter's daily calorie intake.

*   *   *

• A hot dog roll has 108 calories, a hamburger bun, 89. A typical hot dog weighs 1¾ ounces and has 124 calories; a 3-ounce burger (about the size you get at a fast food place) has 140. You get more meat, less nitrites, and about the same calories when you choose a small hamburger rather than a hot dog. Watch out for those giant burgers, though—they're calorie-loaded.

*   *   *

• One ounce of cheddar cheese has 112 calories. If you always thought hard cheeses were a good source of protein, you were wrong. Only about 25 percent of the calories are protein. The rest are fat.

*   *   *

• Turkey yields more edible protein, minus fat or skin, than chicken or duck. You'll get about 46 percent protein with turkey, 41 percent with chicken, and 22 percent for ducklings. (Another reason not to wait for Thanksgiving.)

*   *   *

• Not all processed cheeses are made entirely of cheese. Some processed cheeses have up to 40 percent more water than cheese.

"Cheese food" can legally contain about 44 percent water or milk. Even less real in the cheese section is "cheese spread," which can contain up to 60 percent water, not to mention added gums, gelatins, flavorings, and coloring. Processed cheese food has about 93 calories per one-ounce serving. Cheese spreads have about 43 calories per tablespoon.

* * *

• You have a slimmer chance of being on TV if you're heavy. John J. O'Connor in *The New York Times* noted that while in the real world, "a substantial" number of people are overweight, "the tube world" shows a different picture. A 1979 study revealed that on television, only 2 percent of women and 6 percent of men were fat.

* * *

• Those vibrating belt machines at the gym are about as effective in melting away fat as a girdle is. You have to work muscle and expend energy to lose body fat. You can't lose fat while the machine shakes you up. You're the one who should be moving—not the machine.

* * *

• No comment: "There are certain compensations for overweight women. Men do not suspect them and other women do not fear them as competition." Elsa Maxwell, in her autobiography, *RSVP*.

Chapter 18

The Most Dangerous Things to Put in Your Mouth

Butter

Hey, I know what you're thinking. Everyone knows that butter is dangerous for dieters. Most of us just don't realize how dangerous: 100 calories per tablespoon, and it's a saturated fat. (More on this on the next page.) That calorie count is over twice as high as sugar, over three times as high as bread, ten times as high as potatoes.

A very high calorie count alone is not enough reason to put a food on the top of the danger list. Take cream cheese, for example. The truth is that cream cheese doesn't turn up as often as butter, which goes with almost everything.

I didn't realize how much butter I was eating until my husband decided to total it up. He put a fresh stick on the butter dish before breakfast. Well, I'd put a dab on my diet toast. (Of course, I was dieting at the time.) I used a little on my vegetables and a little more on the fish I broiled. By bedtime, I had used two and a half ounces. That was 530 hidden calories. My daily intake on my 1200-calorie-a-day-diet had gone up to 1730.

Helpful Hints

- Butter the smooth side of Rye Crisp and you'll use half the calories.
- Use whipped margarine or butter. It spreads evenly, so you use less.
- Always cool toast before you butter it. Otherwise, the butter will melt into the bread and tempt you to pile on more.
- Whip your own unsalted margarine. To make two pounds, slowly beat in two cups of evaporated milk (or evaporated skim milk, for fewer calories), a little at a time, to one pound of butter. Pour into bowl and chill.

Fats

Butter has its own category because it's one of the foods that's easy to overdo on. Butter's just a fat, and there are other fats we eat with similar abandon—like nuts, ham, cream, and cream sauces. Fats are also found in meat, poultry skin, dairy products, nondairy creamers, margarines, and salad oils (which are nothing but). We consume about seven tablespoons of fat a day, but the surprise is we only need one tablespoon's worth to maintain good health.

Without some fat, we'd be in sad trouble. You need fat to help keep a sex-hormone balance, and your skin needs it so it won't dry out. Without fat, you couldn't absorb the fat-soluble vitamins like A, E, D, and K.

Fat itself isn't bad, but your fat intake needs watching, specifically fat intake of the wrong sort. Some fats are good guys and some are bad guys.

Saturated fats are the bad guys. A trick to spot them: They're solid at room temperature. Beef fat is one example. In the vegetable kingdom, where most are not saturated, coconut and palm kernel oils are the exceptions. (You'll find these two vegetable fats in some cookies, cakes, nondairy creamers, and sour cream, as well as dessert toppings.)

Polyunsaturated fats and oils are usually liquid and are mostly vegetable in origin. Corn, safflower, walnut, sesame seed, cottonseed, and soybean oils are high in polyunsaturated fats. These are the good guys.

Monosaturated fats, the fence-sitters, are considered neither good nor bad. Olive and peanut oils are monosaturated.

Fats are important to know about for two reasons. They are the most caloric food per gram (9 calories per), and in saturated form, too much can raise your blood cholesterol level. (More on this very soon.)

If you're really into fat follies, you eat fats because they taste good and fill you up. They sneak in all over the place, into every meal. Eat one ounce of bacon fat and you've taken in 126 calories. One ounce of pork fat has 216 calories. If you wouldn't touch organ meat (like liver) but are crazy for pâté, guess what: Eat pâté and you're eating a variety of fat-laden ingredients including chicken or pork livers plus pork meat, cream, egg yolks, flour, brandy, and (often) nuts. The only low-calorie ingredients are the spices. This is why one tablespoon of pâté contains 69 calories (and up) and about 6 grams of fat.

And if you think you're being smart by having half an avocado instead of a fattening meat dinner, you'll not only be eating a food that's 75 percent fat, but adding about 170 calories to your daily intake.

Helpful Hints

- Limit your intake of fried foods or cut them out entirely.
- Avoid cheese dressings on salads. Sprinkle them with lemon juice and spices instead.
- Avoid creamed soups.
- Steam, broil, or poach fish and poultry. Avoid duck or goose, which are very fatty birds. Do not eat poultry skin.
- Trim the fat off meats and buy the leaner cuts.
- Invest in a few nonstick pots and pans. If what you're cooking requires some oil, add a mere drop of a polyunsaturated oil.
- Cut back or avoid nuts (like peanuts) and chocolate syrup, which has saturated fats in it.
- Use low-fat cheeses (usually about 2 percent fat in them) and low-fat dairy products like skim milk, low-fat yogurt, and buttermilk.

Cholesterol

What is this thing called cholesterol and why do we hear so much about it? Cholesterol is critical to life, that's why. We do not have to eat cholesterol-packed foods for our bodies to make use of it—the liver churns out about 1000 milligrams of it a day on its own. Cholesterol strengthens cell membranes and helps manufacture sex hormones, among its other functions. Your liver won't overproduce it, but if *you* overeat the foods that are jam-packed with the stuff, you have problems.

Scientific evidence points to saturated fats and cholesterol as key culprits in heart and blood vessel diseases. Blocked blood vessels are something you do not want. Supposedly, saturated fats increase the amount of cholesterol in the blood, while polyunsaturates reduce the amount. (Monosaturates have no effect.)

Cholesterol has to get carried through the body some way and "lipoproteins" do it. There are low-density lipoproteins (LDL's), very-low density lipoproteins (VLDL's), and high-density lipoproteins (HDL's).

Low-density lipoproteins and very low-density lipoproteins keep cholesterol circulating around your body. Though the bloodstream has "scavenger cells" that get rid of some extra cholesterol, in the course of travel, lots of cholesterol manages to attach itself to arteries—and they clog.

To solve this, you want high-density lipoproteins. These HDL's *(which are increased in number by strenuous exercise)* snatch cholesterol from artery walls and ship them back to the liver. The liver doesn't want any excess and excretes the extra cholesterol as bile through the intestines.

Which foods are high in cholesterol? Eggs have the highest concentration per gram of any food. It's also in meats, whole milk, organ meats, and high in some fish like sardines and shrimp.

Helpful Hints

- The American Heart Association recommends a cholesterol intake of about 300 milligrams or less a day. Invest in a cholesterol counter and check to see how much you're getting.
- Limit your intake of eggs and foods containing eggs. Three eggs a week should do it. Or substitute a product like Egg Beaters, which has about one-fourth the cholesterol of fresh eggs.
- Do not use powdered eggs: They're even higher in cholesterol than the fresh ones.
- Look for hidden eggs in packaged goods and don't discount what you're mixing in batters: they're in cakes, frostings, mayonnaise, noodles, soufflés, waffles, hamburger mix, custard, hollandaise sauce, fritters, pancakes, and even some pretzels.
- Limit your intake of beef, pork, lamb, and organ meats. Eat lean fish and poultry.

No comment (but with respect): The late senator Hubert Humphrey's favorite sandwich was reputed to be made with peanut butter, baloney, cheddar cheese, lettuce, and mayonnaise on toasted bread. And all that with a side of ketchup.

Salt

Manufacturers are legally obliged to list salt on the labels of all processed foods, if they add it at all. The catch is that they don't have to tell you *how much* salt they're sprinkling in. Tricky business.

It sure fooled me for a while. I thought I was being good by not salting whatever was canned or packaged. Little did I know that whenever I ate a processed food, I was also downing a lot more salt that I intended to. Let me tell you about salt . . . and hidden salt.

The recommended daily allowance of sodium is only 1100–3300 milligrams (mg.) a day for adults. A better top figure, according to the American Health Foundation, is no more than 2000 mg. (two grams). Two grams equals a little under a teaspoon. Most Americans use about 2–4 teaspoons a day.

Salt is, chemically speaking, sodium chloride. About 40 percent of salt is made up of sodium. It's the sodium part that concerns you, since a high intake of it has been associated with hypertension, kidney problems, and stroke.

Even if you don't add salt to processed foods you buy, you're probably getting more sodium than you expected in the package. Here's the bad news:

Campbell's Tomato Soup, per 10-ounce serving, has a whopping 1050 mg. of sodium. Take your soup with three Nabisco Premium Saltines and you add another 129 mg. Grabbing a fast lunch? One hot dog on a bun with on teaspoon of yellow mustard and about an eighth of a cup of sauerkraut add up to 1160 mg. of sodium.

If you lose control and binge on one cup of Jello Chocolate Flavor Instant Pudding and Pie Filling, you also get 960 mg. of sodium along with the calories. Eating instant oatmeal at breakfast gives you about 200 times the sodium of regular rolled oats. Cheerios has nearly 2½ times the sodium per ounce of Planters Cocktail Peanuts.

The salt shakers are going strong at the canned vegetable factories, too. Del Monte Whole Green Beans, for one, comes in at 925 mg. per cup.

If this gives you indigestion, don't reach for the Bromo or you add another 717 mg. of sodium per dose. Alka-Seltzer adds 521 mg. and Sal Hepatica 1000 mg. of sodium per dose. Digel's got 170 mg., and while laxatives and some sleep aids may solve some of your problems, they're not sodium free.

And watch out for your water. Yes, plain old drinking water. (Not club soda. You *know* that has sodium.) Some cities have water suplies that are high in sodium due to a "softening process" for hard water. For example, when magnesium and calcium are removed, sodium is substituted.

162

By the way: If you think soy sauce is a smart alternative to using salt, you should know that 2 teaspoons of soy sauce is equal to a half teaspoon of salt.

What about salt substitutes? Though potassium chloride is the main ingredient in these substitutes, other chemicals are present, too. These are used for a variety of reasons—among them, to decrease bitterness and perk up the flavor.

Salt substitutes pose no problem to healthy folks, but the Federal Drug Administration and health experts suggest that if you're on a sodium-regulated diet, be sure your doctor okays any salt substitutes. Potassium (or ammonium) salts can be harmful to people who suffer from certain heart disorders and from kidney problems.

Now, as a sodium-conscious consumer, how do you keep away from the stuff? The words "salt free" on a label aren't enough. If you find the words "sodium" (along with other compounds, such as sodium saccharine or sodium citrate) or "brine," the product may be salt free, but it's not sodium free at all.

Some products are obviously salted. Garlic salt, celery salt, salt pork, and onion salt are self-explanatory. You'll also find sodium in baking powder, baking soda, and self-rising flour. Foods that are pickled or smoked are loaded with sodium, as is any food that contains MSG (monosodium glutamate), a "flavor enhancer."

Remember: The more salt you consume, the more water you retain. As little as three-quarters of a teaspoon of salt can add a pound of weight.

Helpful Hints

- Start decreasing your intake of salt by using spices, herbs, and lemon in its place. Your taste buds can be retrained to like a lot less salt.
- Check with your local water supply company, or American Heart Association, to learn the sodium level in your water. If it's high, invest in a sodium filter for the tap. You cook with that water and make tea and coffee.
- Your library should have a copy of the U.S. Department of Agriculture's booklet called "The Sodium Content in Your Food." (It's booklet number 233.) Check into it to see how much sodium you're getting in raw, cooked, or processed foods. Or, consult *Consumer Reports*, December 1981, for a similar list.

- Buy low-sodium baking powder and baking soda.
- Cut down on processed and canned food and take the time to cook with fresh vegetables.
- Always read the labels on packaged and canned goods. If a product is made with a sodium compound, don't buy it or limit your intake of it.
- Try an interesting tasting salt substitute like "Spike" or "Vegit." Before you use a substitute, check with your doctor.

No comment: Babe Ruth, the legendary Yankee hitter, once downed twenty hot dogs before a game.

Caffeine

In 1732, Johann Sebastian Bach paid tribute to the mighty bean by composing "The Coffee Cantata." The French statesman Talleyrand, a coffee lover, suggested these qualities for a perfect cup of coffee: "Black as the devil/Hot as hell/Pure as an angel/Sweet as love."

Never mind the poetry and music. Coffee's blessed with a zero calorie count but cursed with caffeine. It's also without nutritional value, interferes with the absorption of B vitamins, and doesn't do much for your system. Caffeine is a stimulant and speeds up fat metabolism, but on the other hand, it can cause mood changes, rapid breathing, rapid heartbeat and palpitations, headaches, tremors, and disturbed sleeping patterns. (And you thought you were just in love!) That's not all. Caffeine also causes kidneys to produce more fluid and your stomach to secrete more acid. Researchers are investigating the effects of a substance in coffee on the development of benign breast lumps (fibrocystic disease) and birth defects.

Most teas aren't as chockful of caffeine as coffee is, but some imported varieties sure are. Seems I won't do better with colas, either. Even the one-calorie-per-can colas are high in caffeine count. A twelve-ounce-can of Coca-Cola, Tab, Dr. Pepper, and Pepsi-Cola has between one-third and one-half the caffeine of a cup of coffee. (Plus about eight teaspoons of sugar per twelve-ounce can!) in the non-sugar-free varieties) Now there's a decaffeinated cola, RC 100, which also has one bare calorie, but it's sweetened with saccharine, which, the label tells me, is risky to ingest. If I get a headache thinking about this, I'd better not take Anacin—it's got caffeine in it, too. So do Excedrin, Midol, and not surprisingly, No-Doz.

If you or your kids are lovers of another bean—the cocoa bean—

you can be getting more caffeine than you want in cocoa, milk chocolate, and baking chocolate. Though chocolate has about one-fifth to one-third the amount of caffeine as coffee, it's got a larger dose of another stimulant, theobromine. And chocolate is fattening to boot.

A reasonable dose of caffeine is about 125 mg. a day, or what you'd get in one cup of coffee. At that rate some coffee lovers take in 500 mg. a day and more.

The amount of caffeine in coffee, tea, colas, and chocolate depends on the kind of bean used plus the method of processing, and preparation. How much caffeine are you drinking? *Food Values of Portions Commonly Used*, by Jean A. Pennington and Helen Nichols Church (Harper & Row), cited these figures of caffeine content per 5-ounce cup:

Maxim (freeze-dried): 61 mg. per teaspoon
Taster's Choice (freeze-dried): 59 mg. per teaspoon
Drip ground: 146 mg. per cup with a 137–153 mg. cup range
Percolated: 110 mg. per cup with a 97–125 mg. range
Instant decaffeinated: 3 mg. per cup
Salada Tea: 59 mg. per cup
Lipton (bagged): 54 mg. per cup
White Rose: 55 mg. per cup
Boston's 99½% Caffeine-Free Tea: 9 mg. per cup
Coca-Cola: 65 mg. per 12-ounce can
Dr. Pepper: 61 mg. per 12-ounce can
Pepsi Light or Pepsi-Cola: 36 mg. per 12-ounce can
Anacin or Excedrin: 60 mg. per pill
Midol: 32 per pill
Carnation instant cocoa mix: 13 mg. per package
Hershey instant dry chocolate powder: 10 mg. per tablespoon

Helpful Hints

- Keep coffee consumption down to one cup a day; same for tea.
- Switch to decaffeinated coffees and teas. If you can find them, buy coffees that have been decaffeinated with a water process instead of the chemically treated ones.
- Even better, switch to coffee and tea substitutes. Postum, Cafix, and Pero are all grain beverages without caffeine. They

have about 12 calories per cup and contain some nutritional value.

- Drink, if you must, sodas that are caffeine free. Even better, sip salt-free seltzers or club soda with a twist of lime. You get no overload from sugar or caffeine from these.
- If you're tempted to eat chocolate, remember that not only aren't the fats and calories good for you—neither is the caffeine.
- Send for "Caffeine and Pregnancy," a free booklet that has more information about caffeine's effect on your health, pregnant or not. Write to Consumer Information, Department G, Pueblo, CO 81009 and ask for booklet #612k.

Sugar

A few hundred years ago, sugar was sold in pharmacies. If you got some, it was because sugar was considered more a medicine than a treat. For some of us sugar-holics, it *is* a drug.

It's also delicious. But as TV's "Rhoda" once said about chocolate: "I don't know why I'm eating this. I might as well apply it directly to my hips." A teaspoon of sugar isn't fattening. But for those of us who consume up to 500 calories or more a day from one sort of sugar or another, it's dangerous.

White granulated sugar isn't the only sweetener we down by the bucketful. There's corn syrup, corn sugar, molasses, maple sugar, honey, fructose, maltose, lactose, and for baking, brown sugar and confectioners' sugar. It appears to be everywhere, whether you want it or not.

You know if you eat an Oreo, you're eating sugar. But to comply with America's sweet tooth (cavity-prone), manufacturers add it to hot dogs, breakfast cereals, some processed foods, salad dressings, gums, ketchup, even coatings for food such as Shake 'n' Bake.

Sugar, like starch, is a carbohydrate and a source of energy. A gram of carbohydrate amounts to 4 calories—the same as protein. Simple sugar (as in a chocolate bar) is the quickest source of energy, but it's not long lasting. You get a rapid peak boost when glucose is transported to your cells by insulin, but often your pancreas secretes an excess of insulin and releases more than you need. Your blood sugar drops and you feel worse. To feel better, you eat Reese's Pieces. And the cycle starts again. It's much smarter to eat complex carbohydrates (like pasta or bread) which take longer to get into your bloodstream.

The total amount of calories you eat, not the proportion of calories made up of sugar, is what makes you gain weight. The problem is that sugar addicts can eat a *lot* of sweets—and therefore a *lot* of calories.

If you want to lose weight, sugar's gotta go.

Helpful Hints

- You'd have to eat eight or nine apples (about three pounds) to get the same calories as 5 ounces of milk chocolate. One apple is more satisfying for bulk and sweetness. *Eat fruit!*
- Read the package labels on all foods you buy and check for corn sweeteners, lactose, dextrose, sucrose, fructose, honey, or molasses on the labels. If any sweetener is listed as one of the first three ingredients, the product has a high sugar content.
- Do not keep a sugar bowl on the table. Develop a taste for foods without sugar.
- Increase your use of tangy spices like cinnamon, ginger, cardamom, and nutmeg.
- Don't bake rich desserts or buy any sweets—even if they're on sale. If it's not in the house, you can't nibble.
- Cut down on soft drinks with sugar (they have up to eight teaspoons of sugar per twelve ounces).
- Dried fruits sound promising but they're loaded with sugar. Five dried apricots have the equivalent of about 4 teaspoons of sugar. One-quarter cup of raisins have about 4 teaspoons worth of sugar.

Food for thought: The American Dream: getting rich. The American Nightmare: getting fat.

Alcohol

The only occasion I know of that doesn't "call for a drink" is breakfast. Brunch is close, but no cigar.

Drinking is supposed to make you feel happy, relaxed, a little looser with your words and deeds, social and lots of fun. As we all know, too much booze, and you're on "tilt." There's no fun in that.

Alcohol is an amazing liquid. It's on your food exchange list as a fat, but it's actually in its own category, since it's a drug *and* a carbohydrate. (Alcoholic beverages are fermented from fruits and grains.) When it's metabolized, you get twice the calories per gram as from starch or sugar. It also works on you faster than the proverbial speeding bullet. Ethanol is what makes it happen. Ethanol is an ingredient in alcohol that shoots through your system via your bloodstream. Your liver works like mad to break ethanol down and defuse it, but it can only process so much an hour.

What happens then? Ethanol starts to collect in body tissues. When it hits your brain, you begin to feel light-headed. Give your body a few ounces of vodka (brandy, Scotch) and you're feeling good. A few more ounces and you may trip over the sofa. After five, you're officially intoxicated.

Too much alcohol over an extended period of time can wreck your body. It can accelerate aging (who needs that?), make you forgetful, and cause wide mood swings, to name a few results. You can develop skin sensitivity so great that even a light touch hurts. It can cause problems with blood clotting and high blood pressure.

Alcohol is also very caloric, which is why I'm talking about it here.

One fluid ounce usually equals a shot. The home barkeep may use a jigger, which is 1½ ounces. Think about it. When's the last time anyone served a one-shot drink? Most of them end up being two-shot drinks. Double the calories.

The caloric content of distilled liquors depends on the percentage of alcohol. The proof is twice the alcohol percentage. (80 proof = 40 percent alcohol.) The following values apply to all brands of bourbon, Scotch, rye, brandy, rum, gin, tequila, and vodka.

80 proof 1 fl. oz.: 70 calories	1½ fl. oz.: 105 calories
86 proof 1 fl. oz.: 75 calories	1½ fl. oz.: 112 calories
90 proof 1 fl. oz.: 79 calories	1½ fl. oz.: 118 calories
94 proof 1 fl. oz.: 83 calories	1½ fl. oz.: 124 calories
100 proof 1 fl. oz.: 89 calories	1½ fl. oz.: 133 calories

Let's see what we've got in one glass here (refilled twice). Three Scotch and waters (80 proof, double shots) add up to 420 empty calories. And if you prefer sweet drinks, you're in big trouble. Don't even bring that glass to your lips. Pina coladas, for example, should be outlawed: 6 ounces total 480 calories.

Drinking in moderation is certainly okay. In fact, a 1974 government report said that moderate drinkers are more likely to live longer and have fewer heart attacks than people who don't drink at all, who've stopped drinking, or drink way too much. As far as I know, this report hasn't been challenged.

Helpful Hints

- Don't let two or three drinks (beer, wine, or the tougher spirits) substitute for food.
- Carbonated wines like champagne or drinks mixed with sodas get you higher faster. Those bubbles do it. Straight alcohol is fast, but the carbonation in your stomach makes you absorb the alcohol into your blood faster.
- If you're feeling low, a drink will affect you quicker than if you're feeling okay.
- One drink won't hurt. Choose a lower calorie drink (like "light" beer or white wine or the lower calorie wines) and nurse it.

In case you wondered: There's a trace amount of alcohol in bread.

Diet Pills

When you have a fat problem, what sounds better than a pill that will take it all away? Take two or twenty, and the fat flies off. The truth is that diet pills are about as critical to *long-term* weight loss as the wrist corsage—and a lot more dangerous. The pounds may go, but your health may well depart along with them.

Diet pills used to be available by prescription only. They were called "uppers," or technically, amphetamines. The main reason amphetamines worked was because they suppressed the appetite center in the brain. You just didn't feel like eating. A few problems resulted—psychological dependence, mental disturbances, and elevation of blood pressure. Maybe you weren't eating or overeating, but you didn't feel like living either.

We have progress to thank for a new diet pill that doesn't work with amphetamines, but a chemical that's just as bad. If you're a crossword puzzle fan, you might like to know it's called phenylpropanolomine. This chemical has been approved by the FDA because it's supposedly not habit-forming and it's less likely for a person to become psychologically dependent on it. But a lot of people believe in diet pills. Dieting Americans bought about $200 million worth of the stuff in 1980—Dexatrim, Appedrine, and Control, to name a few brands.

Phenylpropanolomine works like amphetamines. It's a stimulant and constricts blood vessels. Your body takes it as an appetite suppressant. There have been various studies on this over-the-counter "wonder" pill. Pill takers have reported restlessness, irritability, elevation of blood pressure, sleep problems, mental disturbances, and in some cases, seizures and stroke.

There's another reason not to take these pills: Some brands contain caffeine, too—as much in one pill as two cups of coffee. If your heart isn't pounding from the phenylpropanolomine, the caffeine may set it off.

Here's the point: diet pills do not work for long-term weight loss. The brain adapts to the drug and, being smart, soon ignores its messages. The only answer for long-term weight loss is a conscious effort to change your eating habits and attitudes about food and . . . I guess you have my message by now: *exercise.*

Helpful Hints

- Even if you don't feel any of the adverse effects of these pills when you take them, and if you lose some weight because of them, will you be able to keep the weight off? If you're a "yo-yo" weight gainer, the answer's no.
- Don't buy these pills. Don't even read the backs of the packages. They may tempt you.

What would we do without Art: On describing a "powder mix" diet for the *New York Herald Tribune* some years back, Art Buchwald commented, "The powder is mixed with water and tastes exactly like powder mixed with water."

Restaurant Food

Bear with me a minute on this. George Washington once said that the state of New Jersey was a "nest of infamous turncoats." Don't ask me who told me this or why I remembered it, but it sure fits what I'm going to tell you about salad bars. There among the greenery (not in Jersey, but at the salad bar) are stainless steel containers on ice filled with "infamous turncoats"—minced, diced, julienned, pickled, fried, and creamed foods. Think of some of them as traitors, not your pals, and you'll win the war on fat.

I'm not against the idea of salad bars, just what salad barkeeps are shoveling out. What happens to some of us is this: We equate "salad bars" with "as much as you want." Salad barkeeps know they have a good thing going: Their places draw customers. Customers think they have a better thing going because they can pile their plates sky-high.

But do you want to?

Let's take a walk down salad bar lane. You'll usually find:

chopped eggs	green peppers	pickled beets
raw spinach	romaine lettuce	Bibb lettuce
red onions	scallions	grated carrots
Swiss chunked	grated cheddar	bean sprouts
bacon bits	croutons	creamed herring
cherry tomatoes	pickled mushrooms	anchovies
garbanzo beans	Parmesan cheese	olives
pickled herring	Boston lettuce	diced raw zucchini

All this is followed by at least 6 vats of salad dressing and 6 ladles.

One half of this list is good for you; the other half sends your low-cal lunch into the "steak and brew" category not only in terms of calories, but also fat or sodium intake.

Here's the plan; skip the pickled foods, creamed herring, and bacon bits. They're either high in fat, salt, or both. Skip the Swiss and cheddar cheeses and eggs. Pass up the garbanzo beans and croutons and pretend "olive" is only a color. Absolutely do not dip into the Roquefort, French, Russian, Green Goddess, Thousand Island, or any other loving-hands-in-the-kitchen homemade creamy dressings.

So, you say, what's left that's good? For one, your ability to toss a salad that will be filling and still be around 100 calories or so. Your salad will consist of greens, onion slices or scallions, grated carrots, four cherry tomatoes, green pepper, and a mere sprinkling of grated Parmesan cheese.

Helpful Hints

- Don't drop in a "taste" of bacon bits or creamed herring. Cheating is cheating, even if it's by a half teaspoon.
- Mix your own dressing with their lemon wedges and some spices. Ask if they have any low-calories dressings. Better yet, bring your own packets along.

The Continentals

As far as I know George Washington never said anything interesting about French food, but if he tasted it, he probably thought it was pretty *bon*. Who wouldn't? It's a knockout, if you have no weight problem. French food is loaded with cream sauces, butter, and wine; the desserts are to die from, but are they rich!

Italian, Spanish, and German restaurants are not without potential for the danger list—their dishes, too, are made with loads of oil, cheese, and fatty or overly sweet ingredients. Though I'll be dealing with the unromantic side to the French restaurant, follow the same guidelines in Helpful Hints, below, for any restauraunt.

Some dishes appear low-cal but are actually killers in calories. Salmon mousse is one. It's made with eggs and cream. Avoid any "au gratin" dish—that means it's got baked cheese on top. "Cordon bleu" sounds classy, but that means the dish is stuffed with ham and cheese. "Provençal" means it's made with garlic (that's okay) and olive oil or butter (not so okay). "Terrines" will really get you. They're just pâté in another form, made with ground duck and pork plus other high-calorie ingredients. "Pommes frites" are only french fries.

No sauce in a French restaurant is a good sauce—and I'm not talking about the quality of the cookery. Whether it's "béchamel," "béarnaise," or "hollandaise," pass it by. "Vinaigrette" dressing is vinegar and olive oil with seasonings.

Now that you're ready to despair over never entering a French restauraunt again, don't. You can. Look for these key words when you order a dish: "grillade," grilled; "rôti," roasted; "au jus," in its own juice; "au naturel," without any additions, sauces, or tampering with; and "crudités," raw, julienned vegetables without dressing.

Helpful Hints

- When a menu is in another language, ask exactly what each dish is, what's in it, and how it was prepared. If your waiter lifts an eyebrow at you, lift one back. Insist on knowing what you're ordering and don't let a guy in a dinner jacket push you around.
- Request that fish be broiled with no butter.
- Ask that sauces remain in the kitchen, not be spooned liberally onto your plate.
- If dinner comes with fried or heavily buttered oven-fried potatoes, ask for a vegetable side dish (like asparagus) or tiny

boiled potatoes. If the waiter insists there are no substitutions, insist there are. If Princess Di showed up, they'd find some for her.
- Skip any rich desserts and order strawberries or melon in season.

Coffee Shops

Coffee shops are conveniently located, whip up the kind of food you know and love, and the prices are reasonable. However, there's something about coffee shops that immediately makes me think "fat." Maybe it has to do with that open grill. Everything's cooked on it: pancakes, hash browns, burgers, pancakes, eggs, even corn and bran muffins. With plenty of grease.

Sandwiches are usually a big item here: tuna melts; chicken or egg salads; bacon, lettuce, and tomato on white toast. French frying onion rings ruins onions, a perfectly good low-cal vegetable. The cakes are usually about 9 inches high and look as if they're made from spackle and food coloring. The pies, as my friend Roger says, are either blueberry, apple, or cherry "effect." They're so loaded with cornstarch and sugar, you just get the "effect" of eating real fruit pie.

They also offer a "dieter's plate": a scoop of cottage cheese with half a canned cling peach, a burger without the bun, a scoop of cole slaw dripping with mayo, and a carrot curl. Okay on the carrot curl and cottage cheese. You don't need all that protein nor the sugar in the canned peach. You'd actually be better off eating the bun, which you really want and is a source of complex carbohydrates, an appropriate balance for the meal.

There's something friendly about the coffee shop. You want to order friendly foods like salami on rye. But coffee shops are about as concerned with low-cal dining as the French restaurant. It's up to you to say no.

Helpful Hints

- Order sliced chicken, turkey, or roast beef without bread or dressings. Trim the fat from the beef.
- Order "individually packed" cans of water-packed tuna on a bed of lettuce with a side order of tomatoes, sliced.
- Order a baked potato instead of french or home fries.
- Skip the puddings or impossibly caloric desserts. Order half a grapefruit or melon balls.

- Ask them to broil the burgers or broil an open-faced cheese and tomato sandwich instead of frying them on the grill.
- Ask for melba toast instead of bread.
- Ask for sandwiches with lettuce and tomato. These made the sandwich thicker without adding many calories.
- Don't sit around and dawdle. You may be tempted to order a goodie.

Organic, Health, and Natural Foods

I forget the newspaper I once saw this story in, but I like the point it makes. A traditionally minded mother wanted to buy her hip, vegetarian daughter a string of pearls. "Gross," said the daughter, or words to that effect. "Why?" said the mother. "They're organic."

Pearls are organic, vegetables are organic, even mother and daughter are organic. The question is: Are "organic" foods better for you than the commerical "nonorganic" foods sold at the supermarket? Some say yes; others, like me, say no. Good food is good food. If you're smart enough to serve the frozen spinach and throw out the plastic boiling bag, you know the difference between organic and nonorganic.

What's all the flap about organic or "health" foods? So far, there's no legal definition of health foods or of the term "organic." Organic is supposed to describe food that's been grown without pesticides, growth hormones, or chemically based fertilizers when the crop was on the vine. Personally, I'm not mad about eating foods that are coated with pesticides, but the truth is that I don't, and you don't. As it turns out, the FDA has regulations and guidelines about pesticide residues on foods. The amount of these residues is usually infinitesimal.

It is true that most processed foods lose many of their nutrients, and that some foods retain traces of pesticides and are packed with preservatives and additives. But, so far, no one's found any evidence that health foods or organic foods are better for you or any safer.

Organically grown crops are not necessarily more nutritious. A peach grown in California by a commercial producer using chemical fertilizers is as nutritious (more, in some cases) as one grown with manure or compost. What makes fruits or vegetables nutritious, according to *FDA Consumer Magazine*, is the "genetic nature, the climate, the nutrients available for growth, and the stage of maturity at which they are harvested."

174

There have been lots of tests that show that organic foods have little (and often no) difference in taste, appearance, and nutritional value from the commercial product. The biggest difference is—you guessed it—the price.

You may be paying two to three times as much for organically grown fruits and vegetables as what you pay at your local produce counter. Why the cost? Organic farming takes more labor, so for those honest farmers who make a living this way, I can understand the higher prices. The second reason is not so homespun. Because of the trend toward buying organically grown foods, some crooks around are jacking up the price of commercially grown stuff by calling it "organic."

Here's another scoop on health foods. They're often loaded with fat, sugar, salt, and cholesterol. Take the ever-popular granola—it's one of the highest calorie breakfast cereals you can eat. It's got about four times the calories as, say, regular wheat cereal, thanks to the coconut oil (a highly saturated fat) and molasses. Some carob candy bars are made with palm oil—another highly saturated fat. A Tiger's Milk Bar has 250 calories per bar. By comparison, a Nestlé Crunch bar has 138 calories. (Don't buy either one of them.)

If you're on a diet, you may not buy health foods, but what about "natural" foods? Personally, I have no reason to doubt that my Ocean Spray Unsweetened Grapefruit Juice is natural. (It sure wasn't concocted in a lab.) My skim milk Jarlsberg cheese is natural. So is Quaker Oats. How come the companies are hawking "natural" as if real food with real ingredients were just invented? Because it *sounds* so good.

Okay. You buy a food that says "natural" on the label. Sometimes it is. Other times, you read the label and your jaw drops. Right there in black and white, they admit it contains any or all of the following: additives, sugar, salt, MSG (monosodium glutamate), vegetable gums, partially hydrogenated oils, bleached white flour, or food coloring.

Some of the manufacturers say that sugar, white flour, food coloring, and all the other stuff they're dropping in is "natural" or natural enough. (That reminds me of my friend Marilyn, the "natural" beauty, with her nose reduction, chin enhancement, capped teeth, and frosted hair.)

As with organic and health foods, there's no legal definition of natural yet. Generally, it's understood as food that's free of preservatives, additives, and artificial flavors. "Natural" may just mean that the guy at the cheese factory is using real cheese in a product instead of processed; it doesn't have to mean he isn't using some sort of preservative in the prepacking.

You can have 100 percent natural foods, but many items would rot or go rancid without some preservatives. It's not the best news to know your food has preservatives in it, but then again, you're assured of buying food that's edible and safe.

Helpful Hints
- Watch out for "natural" enzymes, "miracle" weeds, or extracts of herbs, beans, or plants that promise weight loss or offer themselves up as food substitutes. I'm talking about, for example, starch blockers (which the FDA pulled off the market in fall 1982) or spirulina.
- Beware those tempting bins of carob-coated raisins and nuts, honeyed dried bananas, coconut chips, and dried fruits. They look tempting, but are high in calories.
- Watch out for "nut" substitutes. They're made with saturated oils.
- Don't buy protein powders, cake or pancake mixes, "protein cookies," or any other product without checking the label to see the fat content (and type of fat), sugar, salt, and other ingredient levels. You may just be getting higher calories at higher cost.
- A slightly shriveled-looking apple at a health food store isn't necessarily a better apple. You're probably better off buying from a reputable produce dealer. Just wash the apple off before eating.
- Read all labels of foods calling themselves natural.
- Send away for a free booklet called "The Confusing World of Health Foods," Booklet #518K, Consumer Information Center, Department G, Pueblo, CO 81009. (Note "free booklet" on the envelope.) You'll learn some more about organic, health, and natural foods.

Cigarettes

I know, this is a diet book. Why am I mentioning cigarettes? Because they're killers, like fat. I know it, but I still smoke. I figure if I could finally lose weight after a long battle, I can stop smoking. That's my next project.

Got any ideas?

Chapter 20

Formerly Fattening Recipes

One way to reduce the calorie count in which you're eating is to add air or water to the food, increasing bulk without increasing food value; the makers of "whipped" butter figured this out a long time ago. Another is by simply cutting down on your portions. In recipes, you can generally reduce the calorie count by decreasing either the fat or sugar content. I use one or more of these principles to adapt recipes for entertaining. I like having company, and I don't think dieting has to turn you into a hermit. It doesn't have to mean dietetic disaster for you or your guests. Look over these recipes for use as is or for ideas to cut calories in some of your favorite dishes.

BRIDAL SHOWER
Pink Grapefruit Punch
Pastel Dessert
or
Strawberry Glazed Cheesecake

Pink Grapefruit Punch
8 1-cup servings/42 calories each

1 10-oz. package unsweetened frozen strawberries
1 liter (4 ½ C.) diet ginger ale
3 C. unsweetened grapefruit juice
mint leaves (optional)

Puree juice and strawberries in blender until smooth. Add ginger ale and stir gently. Garnish with fresh mint leaves.

• Sugar calories are saved by using low-sugar juice, diet ginger ale, and unsweetened strawberries.

Pastel Dessert
8 squares/140 calories each

¾ C. graham cracker crumbs
1 T. margarine or butter
1 C. evaporated skimmed milk, whipped
2 C. sherbet, softened

Melt margarine or butter and mix with graham cracker crumbs, reserving 1 ½ T. crumbs for topping. Pour into 8"-square cake pan. Cool crust in freezer. Chill skimmed milk, bowl, and beaters until almost frozen, then whip. Quickly fold in softened sherbet and spread over crumbs. Sprinkle graham cracker crumbs over top and freeze until firm.

- Thin crust, with reduced fat and no sugar, saves calories.
- Whipping evaporated skim milk (200 calories per cup, unwhipped) saves 220 calories compared to whipped cream (421 calories per cup).

Strawberry Glazed Cheesecake
8 slices/140 calories each

2 T. margarine
¾ C. graham cracker crumbs
¼ C. water
½ tsp. grated orange rind
8 oz. low-fat (2%) cottage cheese
⅓ C. evaporated skim milk
2 envelopes (2 T.) unflavored gelatin
3 T. orange juice concentrate
2 egg whites
⅛ tsp. salt
2 T. sugar
1 C. fresh unsweetened frozen strawberries, mashed

Preheat oven to 400° F. Melt margarine in 9" cakepan or springform pan. Mix in cracker crumbs and press over bottom of pan. Bake 5 to 7 minutes and set aside to cool. In a blender, puree cottage cheese with milk until smooth and chill. In a saucepan over low heat, mix 2 T. orange juice concentrate, 2 T. water, 1 T. sugar, orange rind, and 1½ envelopes (1 T. plus 1½ tsp.) gelatin, stirring constantly until gelatin is dissolved. Remove from heat and let stand at room temperature. In a medium bowl, beat egg whites with salt until stiff. Fold in gelatin mixture and cottage cheese mixture. Pour over crumb crust and refrigerate. When set, add strawberry glaze.

Glaze

In a saucepan over low heat, mix ½ envelope (1½ tsp.) gelatin, 2 T. water, 1 T. sugar and 1 T. orange juice concentrate until gelatin is dissolved. Remove from heat, stir in strawberries. Spread mixture evenly over cheesecake and refrigerate until firm.

- Fat content is decreased by substituting skim milk and lowfat cottage cheese.
- Sugar kept to minimum in crust, cake, and glaze.
- Portions are slightly smaller than traditional cheesecake, which is 320 calories per slice.

FOOTBALL BUFFET
Raw Vegetables
Assorted Dips
Hot Tomato Bouillon
Lasagna
French Bread with Chive Butter *or* Margarine
Green Salad
with Special Vinaigrette Dressing and
Herbed Croutons
Cream Puffs

Bleu Cheese Dip
2 cups (16 1-oz. servings)/20 calories per serving

¾ low-fat (2%) cottage cheese
4 oz. bleu cheese, crumbled
¾ C. plain yogurt
1 T. chopped parsley

Puree cottage cheese and yogurt in blender until smooth. Mix in remaining ingredients. Chill.

Cheddar Dip
1 cup (16 1-oz. servings)/24 calories per serving

½ C. grated cheddar cheese
¾ C. plain low-fat yogurt
¼ tsp. dry mustard
2 tsp. chives, minced
¼ tsp. paprika

Combine all ingredients. Chill.

Hot and Spicy Dip
1½ cups (24 1-oz. servings)/10 calories per serving

8 oz. plain low-fat yogurt
⅓ C. chili sauce
2 tsp. prepared horseradish
1 tsp. minced chives or onion
2 tsp. prepared mustard
⅛ tsp. Worcestershire sauce
2 T. minced celery

Combine all ingredients. Chill.

- Low-fat cottage cheese (200 calories/cup) and yogurt (140 calories/cup) are substituted for sour cream (420 calories/cup).
- Fresh vegetables can include cherry tomatoes, celery, scallions, mushrooms, carrots, green pepper. Have you tried zucchini, cauliflower, broccoli, turnips, beets, and Chinese pea pods raw? You're avoiding the high fat and salt content of crackers when you serve vegetables in their place.

Hot Tomato Bouillon
8 8-oz. servings/35 calories per serving

8 beef bouillon cubes
2 qts. tomato juice

Pour 4 cups hot water into kettle with bouillon cubes; heat until melted. Then add tomato juice and keep on flame until warm.

- This substitutes for high-calorie mixed drinks and gets you just as warm.

French Bread with Chive Butter or Margarine
64 calories per ½″ slice

Use ½ tsp. butter per slice, adding 1 tsp. minced chives to each 4 tsp. butter. Wrap the whole loaf in foil and warm in the oven after you have removed the lasagna and are letting it set.

• Prebuttering the bread controls the size of the portion.

Special Vinaigrette Dressing
1 cup (16 1-T. servings)/30 calories each

3 T. vegetable oil
5 T. wine or herb vinegar
2 T. lemon juice
5 T. water
1½ tsp. Dijon-style mustard
1 garlic clove, crushed
1 tsp. crushed tarragon
1 T. finely minced shallots or chives
¼ tsp. paprika
⅛ tsp. ground pepper
salt to taste (optional)

Mix well in a tightly covered jar. Store in the refrigerator.

• Oil in this dressing is kept to a minimum, and in its place are low calorie extenders such as vinegar, lemon juice, and water.

Lasagna
8 servings/350 calories per serving

¾ lb. extra-lean ground beef
2 garlic cloves, pressed
1 1 lb. 12 oz. can tomato puree
1 6-oz. can tomato paste
½ tsp. fennel seeds
1 bay leaf
1 T. parsley, chopped
16 oz. low-fat (2%) cottage cheese
8 oz. part-skim mozzarella cheese, grated
1 egg, beaten

8 oz. lasagna noodles (about 12 noodles)
1½ tsp. oregano
ground black pepper to taste

Preheat oven to 375° F.

In a large skillet, brown ground beef with garlic and drain off any fat. Add tomato puree, tomato paste, and all seasonings except parsley. Prepare lasagna noodles according to package directions, drain, and rinse with cold water in a colander. With electric beater, whip cottage cheese with egg and parsley. Cover the bottom of a 9″ × 13″ baking pan with half the meat sauce. Cover with half the lasagna noodles, overlapping to fit. Layer with half the cottage cheese mixture, then half the remaining meat sauce and half the grated mozzarella cheese. Repeat the layers. Bake for 40–45 minutes. Remove from oven and let stand for 10 minutes to set.

- This has half the calories of traditional homemade lasagna because we have used no oil, a small quantity of lean meat, low-fat cheese, and a small quantity of tomato paste.
- Fennel seeds help sharpen the taste without the calories of sausage.

Cream Puffs
8 servings/150 calories each

¼ C. butter or margarine
½ C. boiling water
½ C. flour
¼ tsp. nutmeg
2 whole eggs

Filling

4 tsp. cornstarch
2 T. sugar
1 C. skim milk
1 egg yolk
½ tsp. vanilla

Preheat oven to 350° F.

In a medium saucepan, heat butter or margarine with water until melted. Add flour and nutmeg and beat until mixture is smooth and pulls away from sides of pan cleanly. Remove from heat and add eggs, one at a time, until dough forms a thick, shiny paste. Drop rounded tablespoonful two inches apart on a cookie sheet that has been sprayed with nonstick vegetable cooking spray. (You should have enough batter for eight puffs.) Bake for 40 minutes or until puffs are lightly browned, then cool on rack.

Filling
Combine cornstarch and sugar in a medium-sized saucepan. Add milk over heat, stirring constantly, until mixture thickens and bubbles. Beat egg yolk slightly in a small bowl, then stir it into the cornstarch mixture until smooth. Heat two minutes longer, stirring constantly. Remove from heat and add vanilla. Cool.

Preparation
Split cooled puffs and fill with vanilla filling. Optional: top cream puffs with a few sliced strawberries or blueberries, or a slice of peach, pineapple, or banana.

• We cut the calories per puff from the usual 250 calories to 150 calories by reducing the sugar and using low-fat milk.

HOLIDAY BARBECUE
Shish Kabobs
Fruit Salad
French Bread with Herb Butter *or* Margarine
Angel Food Cake with Fruited Whipped Topping

Shish Kabobs
8 servings/300 calories per serving

1½ lb. lean beef roast cubed (3 oz. per diet serving)*
4 green peppers, cut in 1″ pieces
48 cherry tomatoes
24 small white onions
4 zucchini (1 to 1½″ in diameter) cut in ¾″ chunks

---

*You may want to increase the amount of beef for nondieters.

Marinade

2 C. red wine
2 T. soy sauce
2 T. Dijon mustard
½ C. lemon juice
4 T. cornstarch

Mix marinade ingredients and pour over meat cubes. Refrigerate several hours or overnight. To assemble on 8 skewers, alternate meat and vegetables (allowing about ½ green pepper, 6 tomatoes, 4 onions and half a zucchini per portion). Broil on barbecue or in oven approximately 15 minutes, turning once or twice. Baste with remaining marinade during cooking.

- There's very little oil in this marinade, and we've used a very lean cut of meat to save fat calories. Substitute chicken for beef and you save another 100 calories per serving.
- The vegetables accompanying the meat are also low calorie.

Fruit Salad
8 ½-cup servings/75 calories per serving

1 C. pineapple chunks (fresh or packed in unsweetened juice and drained)
½ C. fresh green grapes
2 nectarines, sliced
1 C. melon balls (honeydew, cantaloupe, watermelon, or mixture)
1 banana, sliced
3 oz. (½ small can) orange juice concentrate, melted
¼ tsp. ginger

Toss fruit in a bowl together with a mixture of ginger and orange juice concentrate. Refrigerate and serve.

- Using fresh, unsweetened fruits and orange juice concentrate instead of a honey dressing or heavy sugar syrup saves about 50 calories per serving.

Angel Food Cake with Fruited Whipped Topping
8 slices/140 calories per serving

Angel food cake mix
¾ C. evaporated skim milk, whipped
2 C. fresh or frozen strawberries, sliced, or blueberries
grated lemon rind (optional)

Prepare cake according to package and bake in 10″ tube cake pan.
Cool. Freeze half of the cake and slice other half into 8 portions.
Chill evaporated skim milk, beaters, and bowl until almost frozen,
then whip. Fold in fruit and grated lemon rind. Top each slice with ⅛
of mixture.

- Angel food cake contains less fat than most cakes, so it has 50 to
  100 less calories per serving.
- You save another 50 calories by substituting the fruited topping
  for frosting or whipped cream.

DINNER PARTY
Herbed Chicken
Lo-Cal Twice-Baked Potatoes
Nutty Green Beans
Minted Fruit Compote
Popovers
Pumpkin Soufflé

Herbed Chicken
4 servings/280 calories per serving

2 boneless chicken breasts (about 1¼ pounds each), halved and
    skinned
½ cup chopped green onions
1 T. vegetable oil
1 T. butter or margarine
1 tsp. rosemary
1½ tsp. chopped parsley
⅛ tsp. paprika
½ C. white tuna

In a large skillet, melt butter or margarine with oil and sauté
chicken and onion about 3 minutes. Drain any remaining fat. Add

remaining ingredients, then lower heat and simmer, covered, for 30 minutes or until chicken is tender.

- By removing the skin, using a minimal amount of fat in this recipe, and eliminating high calorie gravy, you keep the calories to a minimum.

Twice-Baked Potatoes
4 servings/80 calories per serving

2 medium baking potatoes, baked
4 oz. plain low-fat yogurt
4 tsp. Parmesan cheese
1 tsp. dried minced onion
paprika

Cut potatoes in half lengthwise and scoop out cooked portion, keeping skin intact. Mash potato, then add yogurt and whip with electric mixer until fluffy. Fold in Parmesan cheese and onion. Place potato skin halves on a flat baking tray or cookie sheet and fill with potato mixture. Sprinkle each with paprika. Bake 20–30 minutes at 350° F. or until top is lightly browned and potato is heated through. (Filled potato shells may be made the day before and covered and refrigerated or frozen for later use.)

- These moist potatoes are tasty and 100 calories less than the usual twice-baked potato recipe, thanks to the yogurt/Parmesan cheese combination being substituted for more fattening ingredients. They also eliminate the need for gravy.

Nutty Green Beans
4 servings/50 calories per serving

2 C. cut green beans
1 T. butter or margarine
1 tsp. lemon juice
1/4 tsp. garlic powder
1/4 C. sliced almonds

Steam beans until just tender. Toss in serving bowl together with margarine, lemon juice, and garlic powder. Sprinkle almonds on top.

- Garlic and lemon juice help spark the taste of green beans without adding salt, and fat is kept to a minimum.

Minted Fruit Compote
4 servings/100 calories per serving

2 C. fresh pineapple
2 medium oranges, peeled and diced
4 tsp. frozen orange juice concentrate
4 tsp. water
2–3 drops mint extract
fresh mint leaves (optional)

Mix ingredients and garnish with fresh mint leaves. May be served hot or cold.

- Fresh fruit and unsweetened juice keeps calorie count down.

Popovers
6 popovers/65 calories apiece

½ C. skim milk
1 egg, beaten
½ C. flour
1 T. melted butter or margarine
⅛ tsp. salt

Preheat oven to 450° F. Spray a 6-cup muffin tin with vegetable cooking spray. Beat milk, margarine, salt, and flour together until smooth. Add egg, beating lightly. Divide batter into six muffin cups and bake at once. After 15 minutes lower heat to 350° F. (do not open oven), and bake about 20 minutes longer until sides of popovers are firm.

- Low-fat milk cuts some of the calories, and these popovers are meant to be slightly smaller than usual.

Pumpkin Soufflé
4 servings/54 calories per serving

Topping

¼ C. evaporated milk
1 tsp. frozen orange juice concentrate
1 C. canned pumpkin
2 egg whites, slightly beaten

1 T. sugar
1 C. skim milk
⅛ tsp. ginger
⅛ tsp. cloves
¼ tsp. cinnamon
⅛ tsp. nutmeg

Make topping first: Chill evaporated skim milk, bowl, and beater almost to freezing. Beat milk until almost whipped, then add frozen orange juice concentrate and complete whipping. Chill until ready to serve. Mix pumpkin, egg whites, sugar, milk, and spices in a blender and divide into 4 small custard cups. Set custard cups in a large deep skillet filled with water within ½″ of the top of the custard cups. Heat water just to simmer over moderate heat, cover, and steam for 15 minutes or until soufflé is just set. Refrigerate until well chilled. Divide topping among four custard cups and serve.

SUMMER PICNIC
Pita Bread with Chicken Salad
Fresh Fruit
Raw Vegetables
Spiced Meringue Drops
Iced Tea with Lemon

Pita Bread with Chicken Salad
Makes 1 sandwich/150 calories per *half*

1 5″ whole-wheat pita bread
3½ oz. white meat chicken, cooked and diced
1 small stalk of celery, chopped
½ tomato, chopped
2 romaine lettuce leaves, chopped
1 radish, chopped
2 tsp. Special Vinaigrette Dressing (see p. 181)

Toss filling ingredients and pack in plastic container. Fill at the picnic so bread won't become soggy.

- Skinless chicken is a low-fat, good source of protein.
- Special Vinaigrette is a much lower calorie substitute for the usual mayonnaise used in a salad like this.
- Vegetables add texture and bulk with minimal calories.

Fresh Fruit and Raw Vegetables

- Take advantage of the season by buying a variety of items that are plentiful and cheap. Serving without sauce and dressing cuts your caloric intake substantially.

Spiced Meringue Drops

30 drops/14 calories apiece

2 egg whites
⅛ tsp. salt
½ C. sugar
½ tsp. cinnamon
⅛ tsp. nutmeg
¼ tsp. ginger
dash cloves

Preheat oven to 250° F.

Beat egg whites and salt until they form soft peaks. Gradually beat in sugar and spices. Drop about 1" apart onto nonstick cookie sheets. Bake 2 hours or until drops are very light brown and crisp.

- Using only the egg white and not the yolk cuts fat calories dramatically.
- These cookies are quite low in sugar.

Alternatives and Substitutes: Or, How to Eat an Egg Without Eating an Egg

I know how it feels to read an article telling you that when you crave a hot fudge sundae, eat half an apple instead. Only a person who's never eaten a hot fudge sundae would be able to say that. There is no appropriate substitute for a hot fudge sundae except maybe a hot caramel sundae. Forget either one while you're dieting. (And remember: No one ever died of a chocolate deficiency.)

There are other foods you eat, though, that you might not be so emotional about. Eating a substitute instead of the real thing might be almost as satisfactory, and you'll save a lot of calories. For example:

• Tonic water adds 99 calories, bitter lemon 144 calories, and sweetened ginger ale adds 102 calories to mixed drinks. Mix all drinks with plain seltzer, which has zero calories.

*   *   *

• Grape jelly, when artificially sweetened, has about 4 calories per two tablespoons. Regular grape jelly is up there at 35 calories for two tablespoons.

*   *   *

• Instead of eating fruit pie (around 410 calories a slice), bake an apple. Flavor it with cinnamon and diet raspberry soda.

*   *   *

• Diet Delight Fruit Cocktail has 50 calories per half cup. Compare that to Del Monte Fruit Cocktail at 170 calories per half cup.

*   *   *

• Schrafft's Light All Natural Ice Milk has 135 calories per four ounces. Schrafft's Chocolate Ice Cream has 165 calories for the same amount.

*   *   *

• Miller Lite Beer has 96 calories per twelve-ounce can. Regular Miller beer has 150 calories for the same amount.

*   *   *

• One Hostess Chocolate Cupcake has 166 calories for a 1¾ ounce treat. Head for the fruit instead. One cup of blackberries has 87 calories; one-third of a papaya, 39 calories.

*   *   *

• Instead of using crackers or melba toast, slice raw zucchini or raw cucumbers into thin rounds as the base for hors d'oeuvres.

*   *   *

• Look for "light" breads (Profile, Fresh Horizons), which have between 54 and 64 calories per slice. (Arnold Brick Oven White has 118 calories, Home Pride Butter Top has 148, and Wonder 100% Whole Wheat has 158 calories per slice.)

*   *   *

• Potatoes are good for you, but you can cut calories even more by eating turnips (or a combination of the two). Two-thirds of a cup of mashed turnips is 23 calories; mashed potatoes, 91. (No butter!)

*   *   *

• Whole milk is actually about 96-97 percent fat free with only 3.25–3.7 percent fat. Skim or low-fat milk has only 1–2 percent fat.

* * *

• Skim milk has 89 calories per cup; low-fat milk about 102 calories; whole milk can vary in calorie count from between 150 and 161 calories per cup, depending on the fat content.

* * *

• Instead of whole milk and whole milk products, substitute: skim or low-fat milk, ice milk, low-fat yogurt, skim milk, buttermilk, and polyunsaturated margarine (about ¾ tablespoon of oil equals 1 tablespoon of butter).

* * *

• Use low-calorie salad dressings.

* * *

• Sour cream substitute? It's possible. Blend one tablespoon of lemon juice and two tablespoons of skim milk into one cup of low-fat cottage cheese.

* * *

• Feed the yolk of eggs to the dog or cat. (They're pretty much invulnerable to cholesterol problems.) Keep the white. Add two teaspoons of polyunsaturated oil to each egg white and beat. Or use any of the cholesterol-free egg substitutes such as Egg Beaters.

* * *

• Instead of cheese, sprinkle bean sprouts on salads. One-quarter cup is only 8 calories and supplies one gram of protein and lots of crunch to a salad.

* * *

• Flavor plain low-fat yogurt or low-fat cottage cheese with an eighth of a teaspoon of vanilla extract. It adds only 2½ calories.

*   *   *

• Love sweet potatoes? Instead, cook up squash. The color is approximately the same, but the calories aren't. One boiled 5-ounce sweet potato has 168 calories, mashed. One same-size serving of acorn squash has about 53 calories; butternut, 88, and zucchini, 46 calories.

*   *   *

• More about squash: Spaghetti squash is a great pasta substitute. Spaghetti has about 200 calories per cup; spaghetti squash only 50 calories for the same amount. You can bake the squash whole at 350° F. for 30–40 minutes, scoop out the seeds, and spoon the pulp from the shell. You'll get squash that comes out as fine strands of pulp that look like fettucini. Add a tomato sauce (no meat or sausage) and season with fennel.

Chapter 21

Seasonal Guide to Dieter's Dilemmas

That word association test (back in Chapter 14, Nibbles) wasn't just for fun. We really do tend to associate names, places, events, and even problems with food. Thanksgiving's not just a time to give thanks, but an excuse to dig into turkey stuffing, sweet potato pie, creamed onions, and apple cider. Christmas? It's a religious holiday, but it's also related to going home, seeing the family, and eating a glazed ham, gingerbread houses and chocolate Santas 'til you drop. New Year's Eve: As much as it's noisemakers, and teary reminiscence, it's also associated with caviar, vats of artillery punch, lobster salad, and an assortment of cheeses.

Let's keep going. Valentine's Day: chocolate, right? On St. Patrick's Day you have a drink or four. Easter? Back to the ham, pineapple upside-down cake, and those yellow marshmallow bunnies. May means Memorial Day and the first outdoor barbecue of the year. June: You're in the mood for a picnic. It's warm, so you bring lots of sugary fruit punch, potato chips, and easy-to-make sandwiches like tuna, heavy on the mayo. July and August, you go to the beach and eat junk food or fry lots of chicken to have around. Labor Day: You celebrate the closing of the season with another outdoor barbecue. October: Trick or treating kids line up for miniature candy bars. You buy a few extra bags, along with candy corn and candied apples. And then you're back at Thanksgiving.

Somewhere in here was your birthday. What's a birthday without cake, ice cream, and a few drinks?

Now, I wouldn't tell you to stop celebrating. You just have to stop making the association between holidays and food so that you are only looking forward to the goodies, not the day. You can start to see holidays as a time to *socialize* with good feelings rather than a time for feeling good from filling up.

How to be a diet-conscious guest in any season:

- When you go to a party or dinner, don't leave the house until you've eaten something first. That's right. Even if you're going out to a dinner, eat first. Have your snack. Otherwise you may start allowing yourself to eat anything in sight with the excuse that you haven't eaten much—plus, if you've eaten, you won't be so hungry.
- If your hostess insists you sample her famous, homemade, calorie-laden whatever, decline graciously. If she further insists, ask her if there's a hospital in the vicinity. When she asks why, tell her you're allergic to the main ingredient and if you eat it, you'll die. It works every time.
- Your diet is your business. Don't tell anyone. Don't even whisper it. You don't want to start a conversation around the table about dieting. You will make yourself uncomfortable. (A few jokers will have a few unnecessary one-liners about fat.)
- If there is a dinner you especially want to go to *and* sample, cut back on calories at least a couple of days ahead of time. If you save up 300 or 400 calories on the cutback, you can have some of Aunt Gert's apple popover delight or an ounce or two of Brie without trembling with guilt.
- If you want a drink, pour a *little* white wine into some salt-free club soda and don't make yourself miserable by preparing all those platters of food you can't touch. Instead, keep busy by arranging flowers, putting out the silver and glasses, or keeping your hostess's kids amused and out of the way.
- Make socializing, and not the food, the focus of the party or dinner. That really is the point, after all.

Holiday Baking and Cooking

- Instead of giving baked good as gifts, make decorations or things to wear.
- If you really enjoy holiday baking, give pies, breads, and cakes rather than cookies. Your friends will notice a cake with a piece missing, but may not be aware that their gift of 3 dozen iced cookies started out from a recipie for 4 dozen.

- Make something you won't be tempted to snack on, like homemade chutney, relishes, or mustard.
- When you mix cake batter and frosting, don't scrape the bowl or pan for the remains. A rubber spatula is a great tool, but when it's got frosting on it, it has a way of looking like a spoon. Don't lick it off.
- Tell your family it's time for a new (low-cal) holiday menu. No creamed anything. No brown-sugar anything. No glazes. No pies. No Grandma's old-fashioned butter cookies.
- If your family wants to take you out for your birthday, splurge on filet mignon (5 ounces, trimmed), one baked potato (no sour cream or butter), a green salad, and fresh melon for dessert. Toast with one glass of wine. Calories: under 500. No birthday cake—that can wait another year.

The author of *Jaws* should know: *Weight Watchers* magazine asked Peter Benchley how he avoided overeating under stress. Instead of heading for food, he told them, he puts on a pair of too-tight pants that he keeps around. This gives him a "firsthand account of what it feels like to grow out of one's clothes. It does the trick," he said. "I lose all desire to eat."

Chapter 22

Other Ways to Fry a Fish

There are better ways to do some of your old cooking chores—ways that help you get the most from food nutritionally and save the most calories. For example, a hint about cooking fish (I didn't really mean for you to fry it—I just thought the title would attract your attention) follows right now:

• If you run a thinly sliced piece of fresh ginger over fish, you'll not only have a lovely ginger flavor, but less of a fish flavor.

*   *   *

• By now you know that if you refrigerate meat soups or stews, the fat solidifies. Since the fat's hardened on the surface, you can scoop it off. You can also skim off the fat while the stew's on the burner. Lower the flame a jot, then carefully put the pot half on and half off the burner. With cooler temperatures on one side of the pot, the fat globules will have less chance to disperse throughout the stew. Result: The fat will accumulate on the cooler side. Be there with a spoon to skim it off.

*   *   *

• When you cook onions, turnips, beets, cabbage, or wild greens, keep the lid off the pot. These vegetables don't like high heat. They react by giving off odors, and becoming slimy and overcooked.

*   *   *

• To preserve the vitamins in carrots when cooking them, cut them up, put them in a smaller skillet with about half an inch of water, cover, and simmer gently. They'll cook quicker, too. The aim is for them to soak up the water in which they were cooking so the nutrients aren't lost in cooking water that is discarded.

*　　*　　*

• Mashing potatoes and pureeing vegetables increases the loss of vitamin C—sometimes up to one-half of it is lost in the process. Cut them into chunks or eat them whole.

*　　*　　*

• Most of the vitamins in vegetables lie just under the skins. Don't pare them too deeply if you *do* pare them, or try to cook them with the skins.

*　　*　　*

• When you steam vegetables, let the water boil before you drop the veggies into the steamer. When steaming, allow an extra 3–5 minutes for cooking than when you use water to cover.

*　　*　　*

• Add butter to veggies when they're hot and toss immediately to distribute it evenly.

*　　*　　*

• Keep the water you've cooked veggies in and use for soups.

*　　*　　*

• Allow margarine to stand at room temperature before using it. Since it's softer, it can be spread thinner.

*　　*　　*

• When you broil meat (lean cuts only with the fat trimmed), don't salt it while it's under the heat. Salt draws out the natural juices.

*   *   *

• When spicing food with paprika or curry, watch the heat level. These spices scorch.

*   *   *

• Haul out the muffin tin, and pop whole stuffed green or red peppers into a section. The tin prevents the peppers from toppling over while cooking.

*   *   *

• Don't use baking soda to preserve the natural color of a vegetable. This just about ruins the nutritional value of the veggie, and adds sodium. Instead, if you're interested in aesthetics, add a drop of lemon juice, which should work just as well to preserve color.

*   *   *

• Don't boil or overcook fruit—you're destroying the vitamin C. Boil water first, then drop fruit in. Turn the heat to low and simmer. Test the fruit so it's not at the mushy stage when it's cooked.

Chapter 23

A Pat on Your (Thin) Back

They say that people like to eat when they are sad, depressed, or angry. If you're like me, you also celebrate with food. You give it to yourself as a reward when you're happy. Do these sound familiar?

> I got a raise. (I'll have a couple of raised doughnuts.)
> My trip to Aruba is on. (I'll make a trip to the deli.)
> My checkup was okay. (See you at the checkout counter.)

This kind of thinking is a no-no, unless you want to keep on gaining like a yo-yo. Stop right now. Reward yourself with anything but food. You'll be saving a lot of money by not eating the way you used to.

- Buy necessities, but make them the best—Givenchy pantyhose, a Dunhill toothbrush, hand-milled soap, a monogrammed washcloth, or a small basket filled with potpourri for the bath.
- Buy a single place setting of china/crystal/flatware—the pattern that you've always wanted. As you reach different goal weights, add to the settings. If you have to lose a lot, here's the advantage: You'll end up with a full service of the most beautiful china, crystal, and flatware in town.
- Treat yourself to the best skin care products on the market.
- Hire a baby sitter for a few hours and browse around the best shops in town.
- If you do your own laundry, have everything sent out once in a while. What a luxury to have a closet full of neatly ironed blouses you didn't have to slave over. Or ironed sheets for a change.
- Subscribe to *Self* and *Fit* magazines. They're wonderful and will inspire you.

- Take a long lunch hour and go to a movie you're dying to see.
- Buy something you think is a real indulgence but one you've always wanted: an electric pencil sharpener, an embosser for your envelopes, personalized stationery.

Chapter 24

A Note About Calorie Counters

I have used three major sources for calorie counts in this book: *Bowes and Church's Food Values of Portions Commonly Used* (Harper/Colophon), C. F. Adams' *Nutritive Value of American Foods* (Department of Agriculture, published November 1975), and Barbara Kraus' *Calories and Carbohydrates* (Signet). There are a lot of other calorie counters on the market—sometimes you can even get free ones from insurance companies—and I would say that most are pretty reliable.

Now don't be terribly concerned about the fact that your calorie counter and the caloric values that follow, or the ones you read in another book, don't always agree exactly. Each one may have minor variations, and for good reason. One is that produce grown (and tested) in different parts of the country may contain more or less simple sugar, depending on growing conditions, so the calorie count will differ. Also, the particular brand of food tested may differ: Whole wheat bread tested by one laboratory may contain different ingredients or ingredients in different proportions than the whole wheat bread tested by another.

The food exchange program in Part Two is designed to help you select foods without having to think about the calories, but I know that some of you would like to have a handy reference for caloric values of common foods. So here goes:

BRIEF CALORIE COUNTER

Apple, 1 medium (2½" diameter)	80
Applesauce, unsweetened, ½ C.	50
Artichokes, ½ C.	10
Asparagus, 1 spear	4
Bacon, Canadian, 1 oz.	45

Banana, medium (6″)	90
Beans, green, 1½ oz.	25
Beef, sirloin or hamburger, lean, 1 oz. after cooking	60
Beet, 2″ diameter, about 3.5 oz.	15
Blueberries, ½ C.	45
Bread, whole wheat, 1 thin slice	40
Broccoli, 1 C. (4 spears)	40
Brussels sprouts, 4	20
Butter, 1 T.	100
Cabbage, ½ C.	15
Cantaloupe, ¼	35
Carrot, 1 whole (5½″ × 1″)	20
Cauliflower, ½ C.	10
Celery, 1 large outer stalk or 3 small inner	10
Cereal	
Bran flakes, ¾ C.	75
Cheerios, ¾ C.	70
Cream of Wheat, ⅔ C.	80
Oatmeal, ¾ C.	100
Product 19, ¾ C.	75
Rice Toasties, ¾ C.	75
Puffed Rice, 1⅓ C.	75
Puffed Wheat, 1⅓ C.	75
Cherries, ½ C.	40
Cheese, Parmesan, 1 T.	30
Chicken, 1 oz., skinned and boned breast, raw	50
Clams, 1 oz.	25
Cornish hen, 16 oz., when cooked, without skin	250
Cottage cheese, low-fat (2%), ½ C.	100
Crabmeat, 1 oz.	30
Cranberries, ½ C.	25
Cucumber, ½	10
Egg, whole	75
Egg, white only	15
Eggplant, ½ C.	15
Flounder, 1 oz.	25
Grapefruit, ½	40
Green beans, ½ C.	15
Green pepper, 1 large	20

Hamburger, lean, raw, 1 oz. after broiling	60
Honeydew melon, ½	60
Lamb, 5 oz. chop after broiling	125
Lemon, 1 medium	30
Lettuce, ½ head	20
Liver, beef or calf, 1 oz.	40
Liver, chicken, 1 oz.	50
Lime, 1 medium	30
Lobster, 1 oz.	30
Margarine, 1 T.	100
Mayonnaise, diet, 1 T.	40
Mayonnaise, regular, 1 T.	100
Melba toast, 1 slice	15
Milk, skim, 1 C.	90
Mushrooms, 4 oz.	30
Mustard, 1 T.	15
Nectarine, 1 medium	35
Noodles, egg, 1 C.	200
Oatmeal, ¾ C. cooked	100
Okra, 1 C.	50
Olives, green, medium, 2	15
Olive, ripe, large, 1	20
Onion, raw, 1 oz.	15
Onion, raw, 1 T.	5
Onion, cooked, ½ C.	30
Orange, 1 medium	80
Orange juice concentrate, 2 tsp.	10
Oysters, 1 oz.	20
Pear, 1 (3″ × 2½″)	120
Peach, 1 medium (2″ diameter)	40
Pepper, green, large, 1	20
Pineapple, canned, packed in water, 1 slice	40
Pineapple, packed in unsweetened juice, 1 slice	60
Plum, 1 medium, blue	50
Pork, 1 oz. after broiling	60
Popcorn, 1 C. (no oil)	55
1 C. (with 4 T. oil)	80
Potato, 1 medium (approx. 5½ oz.)	90
Raisins, 1 T.	30

Rhubarb, fresh, unsweetened, ½ C.	10
Rice, 1 C., cooked	160
Salmon, 1 oz.	60
Scallions, 1 small	4
Scallops, raw, 6 oz.	190
Shrimp, 1 oz. raw	25
Shrimp, 7 oz. canned	230
Snapper, red, 7 oz. raw	190
Sole, 1 oz.	25
Spinach, ½ C.	20
Squash, acorn, 1 small (16 oz.)	160
Squash, zucchini, 6 oz.	20
Steak, 1 oz.	60
Strawberries, 1 C.	50
Sweet potato, small, 1 (4 oz.)	140
Tangerine, 1 medium	40
Tuna, water-packed, 6 ½ oz.	220
Tomato, fresh, 1 medium	30
Trout, 1 oz.	50
Turkey, 1 oz.	50
Veal, 1 oz.	100
Waffles, frozen jumbo (Downyflake or Aunt Jemima)	85
Watermelon, 1 6″ × 1″ slice	100
Yogurt, plain, 4 oz.	70
Yogurt, vanilla, 4 oz.	100
Zucchini, 6 oz.	20

---

*NOTE: Except where indicated, weights for meat and fish are for cooked portions weighed without bone, skin, shell, or fat; meat should be lean and trimmed and skin of poultry should be removed before cooking.

DIET DIARY

Today is _____.

I've been helping myself for _____ days.

EATING

Time of Day	Food	Calories	Time of Day
Breakfast (A.M.)			
Lunch ( )			
Dinner ( )			
Fourth Meal ( )			

WALKING

Warmup (Mins.)	Walking (Mins.)	Pulse Rate During Aerobic Walk	Distance Covered	Calories Burned

TOTAL CALORIES: _____

TOTAL CALORIES BURNED BY WALKING: _____

Notes on today:

Goals for tomorrow:

A Final Thought

You have probably heard of Pavlov's famous experiment. The Russian scientist rang a bell every time he was about to feed his laboratory dogs. Eventually, they came to connect the sound of the bell with the expectation of food, and the ringing of the bell alone was enough to start them salivating. Pavlov called this a conditioned reflex.

That's how some of us respond to the problem of being fat—by conditioned reflex rather than rational thought.

But consider this: Pavlov carried his experiment a step further. He taught his dogs to unlearn their response. He rang bells and *didn't* bring dinner and after a while that sound became a neutral one.

Stop being ruled by the bells.

Index

aerobic exercise, 66
alcohol, 106, 156, 167–68
amphetamines, 169–70
angelfood cake (recipe), 185
appearance, 47–48
apples, 79, 80, 86, 150, 167
applesauce, 89
artificial sweetener, 190
asparagus, 78

bacon, 152
baking soda, 199
balanced diet, 64
bananas, 148–49
bean sprouts, 192
beans, 80
  green (recipe), 186
beet greens, 79
beets, 155
behavioral techniques, 121–136
between-meal eating, 123–24
binges, 52, 123, 143
body fat, 58, 61–62, 147, 148
bouillon, 154
  tomato (recipe), 180
breads, light, 191
broccoli, 84
broth, 154
brown fat, 58
buffet (recipes), 179–83
butter, 149, 158

caffeine, 164–65
calcium, 154–55
calorie counter, 202–5
calories, 62
  adding, 90
  reduced vs. low, 146
  use of, 39

cantaloupes, 75
carbohydrates, 58, 64, 146
carrots, 78, 83, 84, 85, 155, 197
celery, 150
cellulite, 42
cereal, cooked, 84
cheese
  Brie, 154
  cheddar, 156
  cottage, 192
  processed, 156–57
cheese cake, strawberry glazed
    (recipe), 178
chicken, 75, 85, 156
  herbed (recipe), 185–86
  salad (recipe), 188
chocolate, 166
cholesterol, 160–61
cigarettes, 176
clothes, 48, 51, 122, 130
cocoa, 164–65
coffee, 164
coffee substitutes, 165–66
consommé, 154
cooking, for family, 49
cottage cheese, 192
crash diets, 30, 47
cravings, 122–23
cream, nondairy, 150–51
cream puffs (recipe), 182
cucumbers, 75
curry, 198

dessert (recipes), 178–79, 182,
    184–85, 187, 189
diets
  1000-calorie, 67–89
  1200-calorie, 91
  selecting own, 90–106

diet diary, 52, 68, 122
diet fads, 8–12, 33, 59–61
diet pills, 169–70
dinner party (recipes), 185–89
dips (recipes)
  bleu cheese, 179
  cheddar, 180
  hot and spicy, 180
duck, 156

eating techniques, 121–136
eggnog, 139
eggplant, 150
eggs, 75, 192
  scrambled, 79
  hard-boiled, 80
  poached, 88
ego boosts, 200–1
energy, 59–60, 124
exercise, 38–44, 66, 147; see also
  walking
exercise machines, 157

fad diets, 8–12, 33, 59–61
fast foods, 139–43
fat cells, 58, 61–62, 147, 148
fat content, 39
fat loss program, 64
fats, 61–62, 159–60
  equivalencies, 104–5
fiber, 155
fish, 76, 145, 197
food intake, increasing, 61
fourteen-day menu plan, 72–89
french bread, 181
french fried potatoes, 141
fruit, 84, 167
  cocktail, 190
  compote (recipe), 187
  cooking, 199
  equivalencies, 94-96

salad (recipe), 184
fruits, dried, 167

genes, 57–58
gift baking, 195
ginger, fresh, 197
goal weight, 51, 68
granola, 175
grapefruit, 82, 148
gum, 139–40, 146–47

habits, changing, 66; see also
  behavioral techniques
hamburgers, 156
health clubs, 134–35
health food, 174–76
heart rates, 112
Help Yourself Diet, 67–89
heredity, 57–58
hints, 73
holiday barbecues (recipes),
  183–85
holidays, 194–96
honey, 153
hot dogs, 156

ice cream, 153

jelly, 190
jogging, 41–42, 108–9

labels, reading, 129–30, 167
lasagna (recipe), 181–82
lecithin, 151
leftovers, 36, 73
lettuce, 76
lipoproteins, 160–61

maintaining weight, 52
margarine, 149–50, 198
marinade (recipe), 184
meals, frequency of, 65, 123

measurements, 126
meat, 73, 144–45, 153
  broiling, 198
  equivalencies, 99–103
  stew (recipe), 197
menus, choosing, 90–106
meringue drops (recipe), 189
metabolism, 34, 35, 58, 60, 61, 66
milk, 154, 191–92
  equivalencies, 94
  varieties, 94, 146
mints, 156
multivitamins, 68
muscles, 39, 42, 60, 63, 64, 66
mushrooms, 73, 80, 81

natural foods, 174–76
natural weight, 59
noncaloric foods, 105–6
nutrition, 132
nuts, 155

orange juice concentrate, 81
oranges, 80
organic foods, 174–76

paprika, 88, 198
parsley, 75
parties, 47, 195
peaches, peeling, 85
peanut butter, 141–42
peanuts, 153
peppers, cooking, 199
phenylpropanoline, 170
photographs, during diet, 125–26
picnics (recipes), 188–89
pie, 155–56
pinch test, 63
pineapples, 148
pizza, 142

popcorn, 139
popovers (recipe), 186
potatoes, 86, 191, 198
  baked (recipe), 186
poultry, 155
procrastination, 121–22
pulse rate, taking, 111–12
pumpkin soufflé (recipe), 187–88
punch (recipe), 177

radishes, 155
raisins, 84
recipes, 177–89
restaurant food, 131–32, 170–71
  coffee shops, 173–74
  foreign, 172–73
rice, 148

salad dressing, 80
salads, 171
salt, 154, 161–64
salt substitutes, 163
scales, 62–63
  food, 127
self-analysis, 126–28
serotonin, 58
setpoint, 34–35, 59
sherbet, 153
sherry, cooking, 153
shish kabob (recipe), 183–84
shopping, 36, 128–30
shopping list, 69–71
shrimp, 78
  canned, 83, 87
snacks, 73, 75, 139–40
soft drinks, 164, 166
sour cream substitutes, 192
spaghetti, 193
spaghetti squash, 193
spices, 81, 141
splurges, 196
spot reducing, 42

squash, 192
starches, equivalencies, 96–99
stomach shrinking, 150
strawberries, 76, 86, 87
sweeteners, artificial, 75
substitutions, 190–93
sugar, 153, 166–67
sugarless foods, 146–47
"sugar-free" foods, 149
sweet potatoes, 88, 192

taste buds, 142
teas, 164
thermogenesis, 65, 66
tofu, 146
tomatoes, 76, 86, 87
tonic water, 190
Triscuits, 155
tuna fish, 77, 152–53
turkey, 152, 156
turnips, 191

vegetable oils, 150
vegetables, 155
cooking, 197–99

equivalencies, 103–4
steamed, 154
vinaigrette (recipe), 181

yogurt, 75, 153, 192
frozen, 154

walking, 40–44, 107–20
amount, 110
benefits, 119–20
cassettes, 118
clothes, 117
distance, 113
equipment, 118
frequency, 110
program, 110–20
footwear, 117
speed, 111–113
time of day, 110–11
warmup exercises, 114–15
weather, 116–17
water, 68, 162, 163
weighing, 127